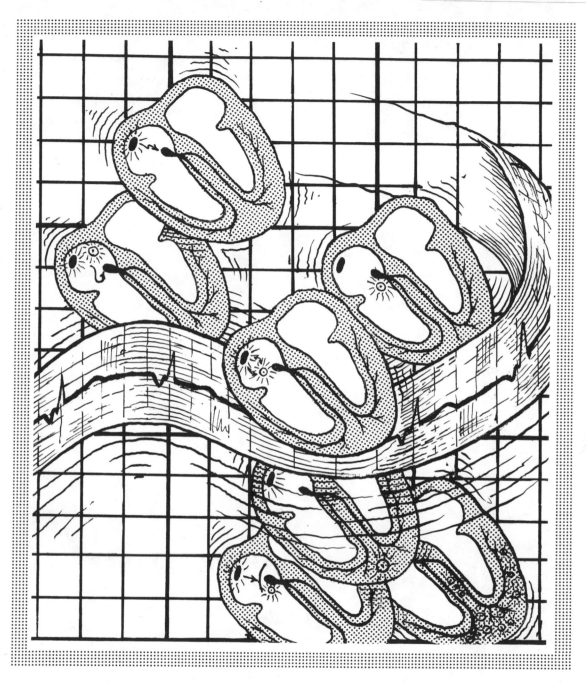

INTERPRETATION of ARRHYTHMIAS
A Self-Study Program

INTERPRETATION of ARRHYTHMIAS

A SELF-STUDY PROGRAM

EMANUEL STEIN, M.D., M.P.H.
F.A.C.P., F.A.C.C., F.C.C.P.

Associate Dean and Director, Eastern
Virginia Graduate School of Medicine

Professor of Internal Medicine and

Professor of Family and Community Medicine,
Eastern Virginia Medical School,
Norfolk, Virginia

Medical Director, United States Public
Health Service, Ret.

Diplomate, American Board of Internal
Medicine and Subspecialty Board of
Cardiovascular Disease

Illustrations by
THOMAS XENAKIS, M.A., A.M.I.

Lea & Febiger   1988   Philadelphia

Lea & Febiger
600 Washington Square
Philadelphia, Pa 19106-4198
U.S.A.
(215) 922-1330

Library of Congress Cataloging-in-Publication Data

Stein, Emanuel,
    Interpretation of arrhythmias.

    Includes index.
    1. Arrhythmia—Programmed instruction.   I. Title.
[DNLM: 1. Arrhythmia—programmed instruction.   2. Elec-
trocardiography—programmed instruction. WG 18 S819i]
RC685.A65S75   1988   616.1'28'077   87-32423
ISBN 0-8121-1143-5

PRINTED IN THE UNITED STATES OF AMERICA

Print No.   5   4   3   2   1

TO THE MEMBERS OF THE HEALTH PROFESSIONS

who will benefit from this effort
and from whom I continue to learn

Preface

Heart rhythm disturbances remain under intensive investigation. The establishment of coronary care units and advances in diagnosis and therapy continue to give great impetus to this study. It is vital for members of the health professions caring for patients with abnormal heart rhythms to be able to recognize the common arrhythmias. This book is simply written and graphically illustrated to provide a firm foundation with a step-by-step approach. After you have learned the basic arrhythmias and have completed all the exercises and practice rhythm analyses, the book can serve as a study guide as well as a teaching, reference, and review manual. When using the program as a review, one can cover the basic arrhythmias in one sitting.

The book is divided into seven chapters. The first two chapters introduce basic cardiac electrophysiology, identification of waves, intervals and segments, determination of heart rate and principal measurements. Normal sinus rhythm and sinus rhythm alterations, atrial, junctional and ventricular arrhythmias, as well as atrioventricular conduction disturbances, are studied in the remaining chapters.

At the end of each of the last five chapters are practice rhythms for analysis related to that chapter. The analyses follow the practice rhythms. At the end of the book is a series of rhythms relating to all the chapters for practice and review. Here, too, the analyses follow the practice rhythms. It is hoped that you will be stimulated to continue learning about arrhythmias and progress to the complete, 12-lead electrocardiogram using the vector approach.[1] This will permit you to recognize other abnormal states such as hypertrophy, ventricular repolarization abnormalities, myocardial infarction and intraventricular conduction disturbances.

I have had the opportunity of reaching thousands of people during my decades in medical practice and tens of thousands more through my books and courses. If I have made life and learning easier I shall treasure it as a major accomplishment of my lifetime.

I thank Mr. R. Kenneth Bussy, Mr. Samuel Rondinelli, Ms. Dorothy DiRienzi, and Ms. Tanya Lazar of Lea & Febiger for their help in making this book possible, and Mr. Thomas Xenakis for elegantly translating my drawings. I add my appreciation to Dr. William Fox[2], Dr. David B. Propert, and Dr. Donald W. Drew for providing electrocardiograms that have enriched this work.

Norfolk, Virginia   Emanuel Stein, M.D.

---

[1] Stein, E.: Clinical Electrocardiography, A Self-Study Course, Philadelphia, Lea & Febiger, 1987.
[2] Fox, W. and Stein, E.: Cardiac Rhythm Disturbances, A Step-by-Step Approach, Philadelphia, Lea & Febiger, 1983.

Contents

Chapter 1

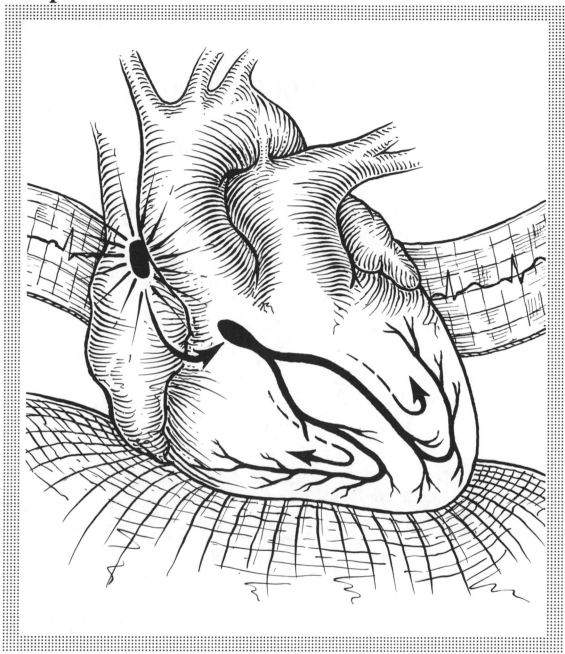

Cardiac Electrophysiology
Basic Concepts

The Electrocardiogram

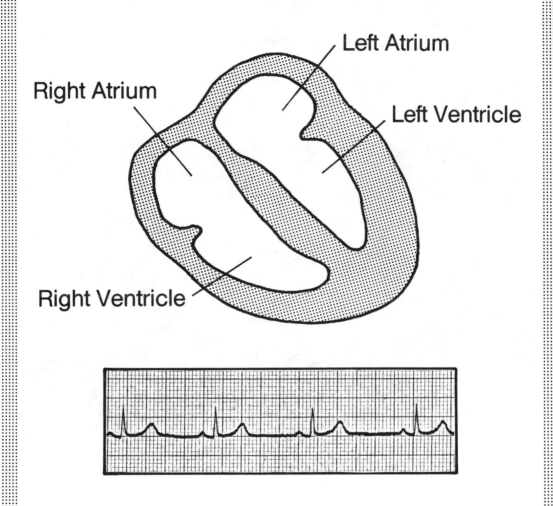

The electrocardiogram (abbreviated ECG) is a recording of the electrical activity of the heart from the body surface. By the placement of electrodes on designated areas of the body, we usually record various views of this electrical activity. All four chambers, the left and right atria and the left and right ventricles, are represented on this recording. Willem Einthoven, who contributed greatly to early electrocardiography, is often called the father of electrocardiography.

Depolarization and Repolarization

(+)　(+)　(+)　(+)　(+)　(+)　(+)　(+)　(+)　(+)　(+)　(+)　(+)　(+)　(+)
(-)　(-)　(-)　(-)　(-)　(-)　(-)　(-)　(-)　(-)　(-)　(-)　(-)　(-)　(-)

Cardiac Cell

(-)　(-)　(-)　(-)　(-)　(-)　(-)　(-)　(-)　(-)　(-)　(-)　(-)　(-)　(-)
(+)　(+)　(+)　(+)　(+)　(+)　(+)　(+)　(+)　(+)　(+)　(+)　(+)　(+)　(+)

1. Resting or Polarized State

(-)　(-)　(-)　(-)　(-)　(-)　(-)　(-)　(-)　(-)　(+)　(+)　(+)　(+)
(+)　(+)　(+)　(+)　(+)　(+)　(+)　(+)　(+)　(+)　(+)　(-)　(-)　(-)　(-)

(+)　(+)　(+)　(+)　(+)　(+)　(+)　(+)　(+)　(+)　(+)　(-)　(-)　(-)　(-)
(-)　(-)　(-)　(-)　(-)　(-)　(-)　(-)　(-)　(-)　(+)　(+)　(+)　(+)

2. Depolarization, Almost Complete

(-)　(-)　(-)　(+)　(+)　(+)　(+)　(+)　(+)　(+)　(+)　(+)　(+)　(+)　(+)
(+)　(+)　(+)　(-)　(-)　(-)　(-)　(-)　(-)　(-)　(-)　(-)　(-)　(-)　(-)

(+)　(+)　(+)　(-)　(-)　(-)　(-)　(-)　(-)　(-)　(-)　(-)　(-)　(-)　(-)
(-)　(-)　(-)　(+)　(+)　(+)　(+)　(+)　(+)　(+)　(+)　(+)　(+)　(+)　(+)

3. Repolarization, Almost Complete

The function of the heart is to pump blood for the body's needs. The *mechanical* act of pumping blood is preceded by, and responsive to, an *electrical* stimulus. The electrocardiogram is a recording of these electrical events. In order for current to flow, there must be *positive* (+) and *negative* (−) charges. These are contained in and around the specialized cells of the heart. In the resting state the outside of the cell is more positive relative to the inside of the cell. This is the balanced or *polarized* state, with no flow of electricity. When the polarized cell is stimulated, the polarity

Physiologic Properties of Myocardial Cells

Automaticity -

Ability to Initiate an Impulse

———

Excitability -

Ability to Respond to an Impulse

———

Conductivity -

Ability to Transmit an Impulse

———

Contractility -

Ability to Respond with Pumping Action

of the cell is reversed. The inside of the cell becomes more positive relative to the outside. This process is known as *depolarization* and reflects the flow of an electrical current to all cells along the pathways of conduction. The cell then returns to its original resting state by the process called *repolarization*. The physiologic properties of myocardial cells permitting these events to occur and leading to contraction of the heart muscle are listed above.

Electrical Conduction System of the Heart

Bundle of His

Right Atrium   **Left Atrium**

SA Node

Left Bundle Branch

AV Node

Right Bundle Branch

Right Ventricle

Left Ventricle

Purkinje System

The processes just described follow specific pathways within the heart known as its electrical conduction system. The *sinoatrial (SA) node* is normally the site of origin of the electrical impulse, leading to depolarization of the atria. The impulse then spreads through the *atrioventricular (AV) node* and *bundle of His* to the *left (LBB)* and *right (RBB) bundle branches* and then to the ventricles through the *Purkinje fiber network,* leading to ventricular depolarization.

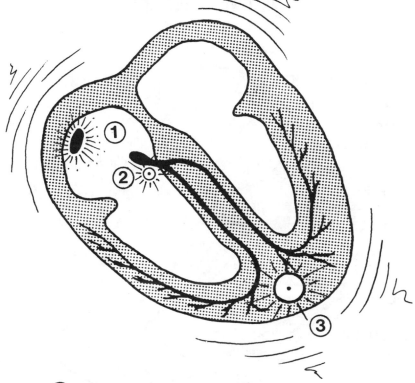

Rate of Impulse Formation
(Impulses Per Minute)

① SA Node   60-100

② AV Junction 40-60

③ Ventricle   20-40

Although the primary and dominant pacemaker of the heart is the *SA node,* under various circumstances and stimuli, another pacemaker may become dominant. There may be two or more pacemakers propagating impulses at the same time. Each pacemaker has its own *inherent rate.* In general, the pacemaker with the fastest inherent rate becomes the dominant cardiac pacemaker. The SA node emits from 60 to 100 impulses per minute, the AV junction from 40 to 60 impulses per minute and still lower pacemakers, such as a ventricular pacemaker, from 20 to 40 impulses per minute. Thus, the SA node is usually the fastest and dominant cardiac pacemaker. If a secondary pacemaker, such as the junctional or ventricular pacemaker, speeds up, it may become the dominant pacemaker. Also, if the SA node slows down or fails, a secondary pacemaker may become dominant.

Autonomic Nervous System Sympathetic and Parasympathetic Nerves

Sympathetic System
- Supplying both Atria and Ventricles

Mediator - Norepinephrine

Increases:
Rate of SA Node
Rate of Atrioventricular Conduction

Excitability

Force of Contraction

Parasympathetic System (Vagus Nerve)
- Supplying Atria Primarily

Mediator - Acetylcholine
Decreases:
Rate of SA Node
Rate of Atrioventricular Conduction
Excitability

The heart is also influenced by both branches of the autonomic nervous system, the *sympathetic* and *parasympathetic nerves*. Stimulation of the sympathetic system, supplying both atria and ventricles, with norepinephrine as the mediator, leads to increased rate of the SA node, increased atrioventricular conduction, increased excitability and increased force of contraction. Stimulation of the parasympathetic system (vagus nerve), supplying primarily the atria, with acetylcholine as the mediator, leads to decreased rate of the SA node, decreased atrioventricular conduction and decreased excitability. If one system is blocked, the effects of the other are seen. For example, if the sympathetic system were blocked, the effects of the parasympathetic system would be elicited.

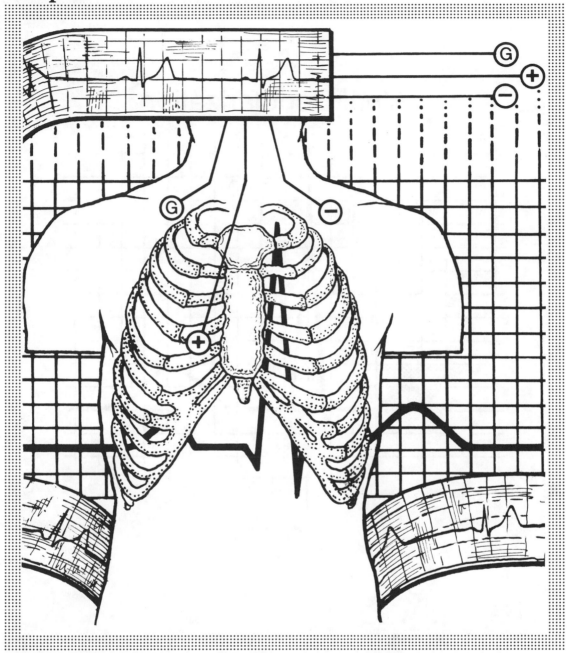

Chapter 2

Electrocardiographic Waves, Intervals and Segments; Lead Placement in Rhythm Analysis; Determination of Heart Rate, PR and QRS Intervals

Atrial Depolarization

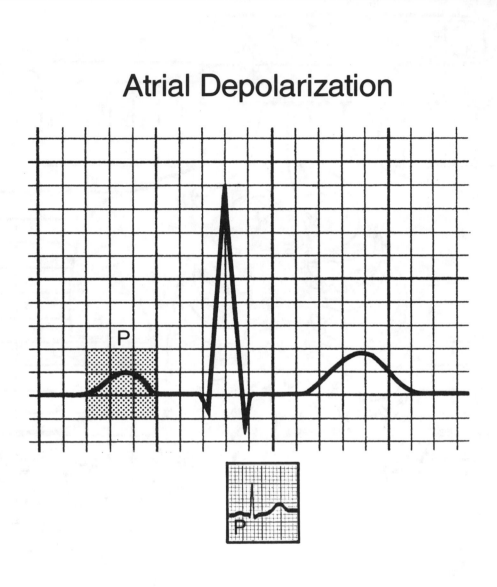

The wave of depolarization that begins in the SA node spreads to both atria, first to the right atrium, then to the left atrium. The depolarization of both atria is represented by the *P wave* on the electrocardiogram. The P wave is normally the first electrocardiographic deflection of each cardiac cycle.

PR Segment

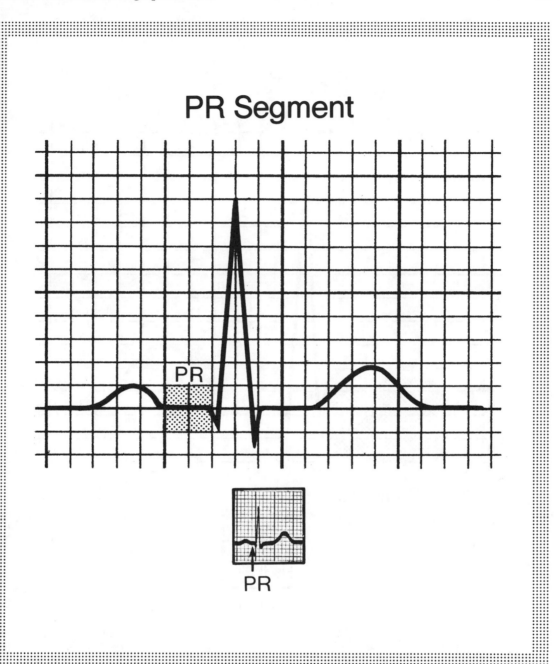

During the *PR segment*, following atrial depolarization, the electrical impulse spreads to the AV node, bundle of His and bundle branches. In the specialized electrophysiology laboratory, recordings can be made from the bundle of His using special recording techniques. On the clinical electrocardiogram, only the flat line is generally seen.

PR Interval

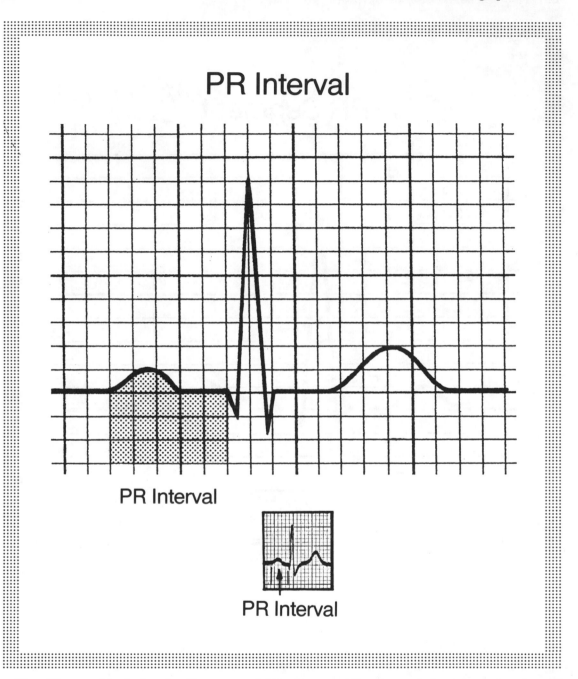

The *PR interval* includes the P wave and PR segment. The interval represents the time of transmission of the electrical impulse from the atria to the ventricles.

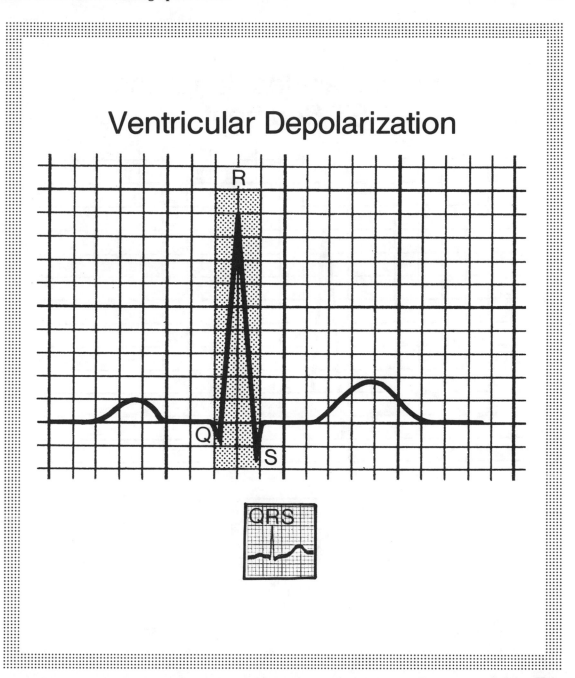

Depolarization of both ventricles is reflected in the *QRS complex.* The *R wave* is the initial positive deflection (upward, above the resting baseline of the electrocardiogram) of the QRS complex. The negative deflection (downward, inverted, occurring below the resting baseline of the electrocardiogram) *before* the R wave is the *Q wave.* The negative deflection *after* the R wave is the *S wave,* which is usually the terminal part of the QRS complex.

Ventricular Repolarization
ST Segment

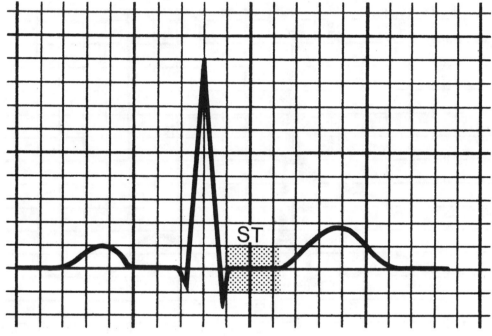

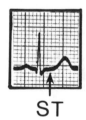

ST

The *ST segment* extends from the end of the QRS complex to the beginning of the T wave (see next page). It represents the earlier phase of repolarization of both ventricles. The ST segment is normally isoelectric (at the same level as the resting baseline). It is neither elevated (positive) nor depressed (negative). The point at which the ST segment joins the QRS complex is known as the J (for junction) point.

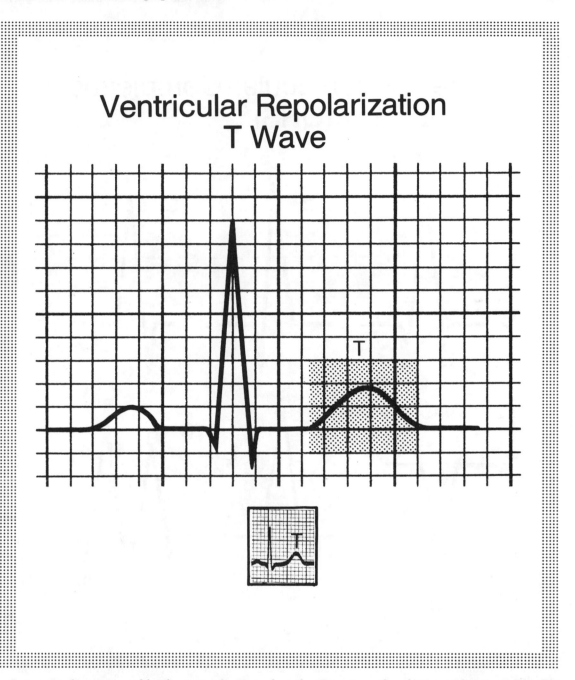

Ventricular Repolarization
T Wave

Later repolarization of both ventricles inscribes the *T wave* on the electrocardiogram. The ST segment and the T wave are sensitive indicators of the status of the ventricular myocardium. *Atrial repolarization* is not often seen on the electrocardiogram because of its small size and because it coincides with the QRS complex.

Types of Ventricular Complexes (QRS)*

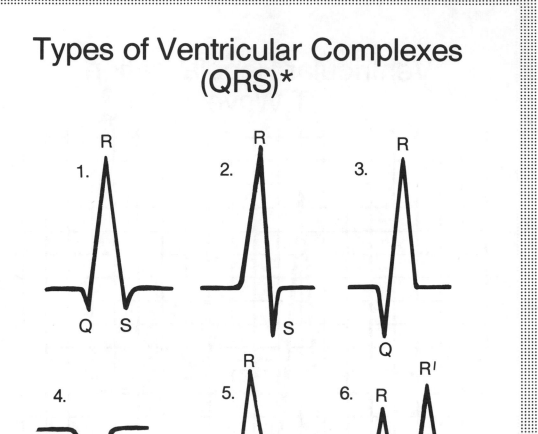

1. QRS; Q wave—negative deflection before the R wave
     R wave—positive deflection
     S wave—negative deflection after the R wave
2. RS; no Q wave present
3. QR; no S wave present
4. QS; totally negative complex, no R wave present
5. R; no Q or S waves present
6. QRSR′S′, a second positive deflection after an S wave is an R′ (R prime), which, in turn, may be followed by a second negative deflection, an S′ (S prime).

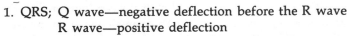

*Although not all of the ventricular complexes contain Q, R, and S waves, they are still commonly called QRS complexes.

Practice

Identify the Principal Electrocardiographic Waves (P, QRS and T)

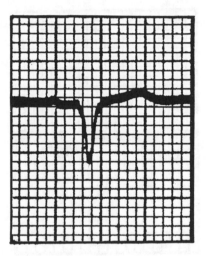

Answer:

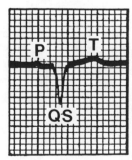

Remember:
    The Q wave is ALWAYS negative
    The R wave is ALWAYS positive
    The S wave is ALWAYS negative
The P and T waves may be positive or negative. When there is no R wave, only one large negative wave, it is called a QS wave, as above.

Practice

Identify the Principal Electrocardiographic Waves (P, QRS and T)

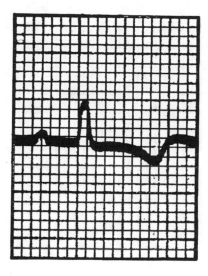

Answer:

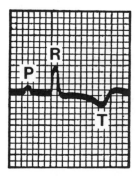

Note again: Although not all of the ventricular complexes contain Q, R, and S waves, they are commonly called QRS complexes. Here, the P wave is positive and the T wave is negative.

Practice

Identify the Principal Electrocardiographic Waves (P, QRS and T)

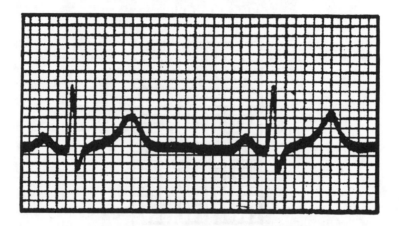

Answer:

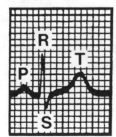

This ventricular complex contains an R wave (positive) and an S wave (negative).

Practice

Identify the Principal Electrocardiographic Waves (P, QRS and T)

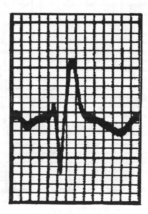

Answer:

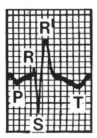

This ventricular complex begins with a small positive deflection, the R wave, followed by a negative deflection, the S wave, then another positive deflection, the R' wave. Both the P and T waves are negative in this lead.

Practice

Identify the Principal Electrocardiographic Waves (P, QRS and T)

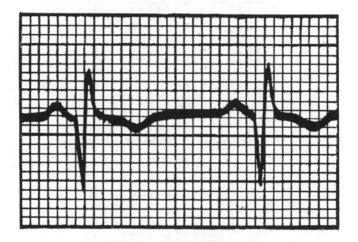

Answer:

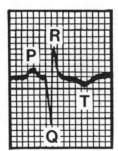

The ventricular complex is initiated by a negative deflection, the Q wave, followed by an R wave. The T wave is negative.

Practice

Identify the Principal Electrocardiographic Waves (P, QRS and T)

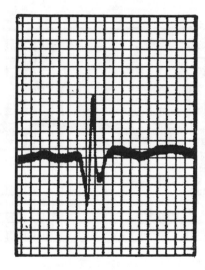

Answer:

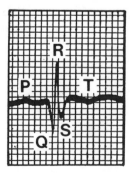

The three components of the QRS complex are seen here—the Q, R, and S waves.

Summary

Electrocardiographic Waves, Intervals and Segments

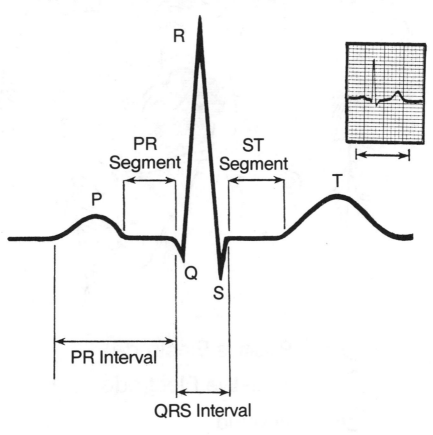

Thorough familiarity with the nomenclature of the components of the cardiac cycle is vital in electrocardiography. Prior to studying the placement of the leads, heart rate determination, and measurements, review all the material studied so far.

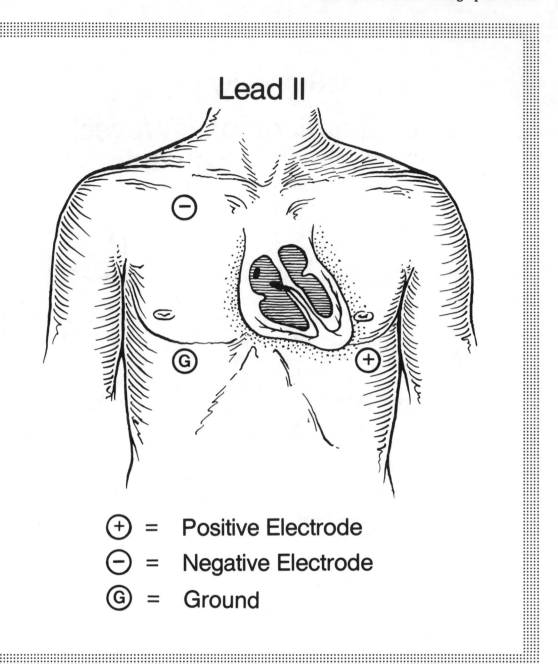

Lead II

⊕ = Positive Electrode

⊖ = Negative Electrode

Ⓖ = Ground

In order for electrical current to flow, there must be a positive and a negative electrode forming a *lead*. Various leads many be used in monitoring arrhythmias, with each lead "looking" at the heart from a different vantage point. A common lead used is *lead* II (two), as illustrated above.

Please note: The complete electrocardiogram consists of 12 leads. To monitor arrhythmias, however, a single lead is generally used.

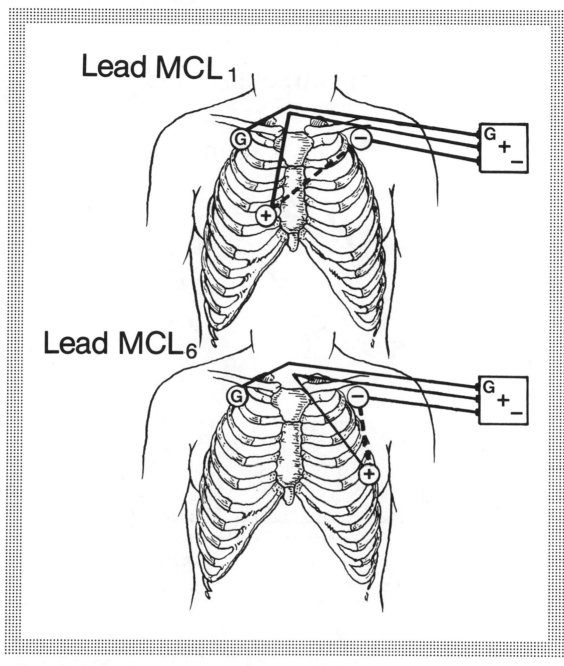

Lead MCL$_1$

Lead MCL$_6$

Two other leads commonly used to monitor arrhythmias are the modified chest leads *MCL$_1$* and *MCL$_6$* as illustrated above.

Heart Rate

Paper Speed = 25 mm./sec.

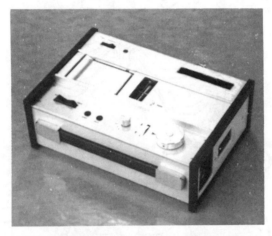

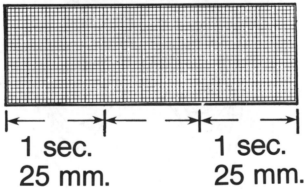

← 1 sec. →	← 1 sec. →
1 sec.	1 sec.
25 mm.	25 mm.

The determination of heart rate from the electrocardiogram depends on the speed of the paper when recording the electrocardiogram. The standard speed of the paper is *25 mm. (five large boxes) per second.* Whenever the paper speed is changed, which is possible on most machines, it should be indicated on the electrocardiogram.

Heart Rate

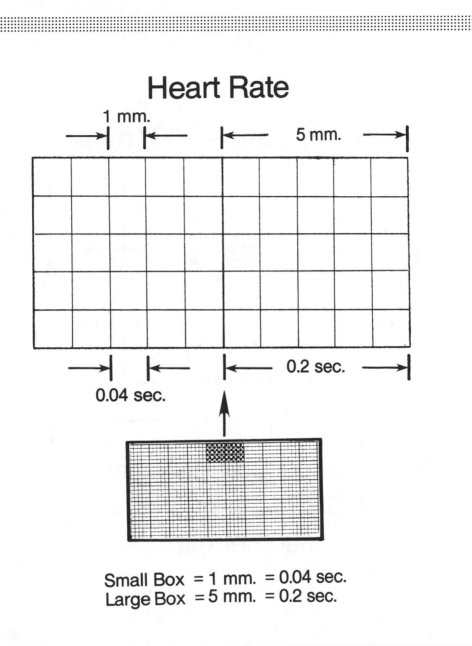

Small Box = 1 mm. = 0.04 sec.
Large Box = 5 mm. = 0.2 sec.

The electrocardiogram is recorded on lined paper that consists of large and small boxes. *Each large box measures 5 mm.* and *each small box 1 mm.* At the paper speed of 25 mm. per second, *each large box represents 0.2 second* and *each small box 0.04 second.*

Heart Rate = 300/min.

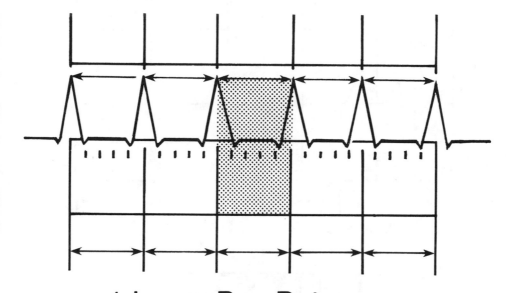

1 Large Box Between
2 QRS Complexes =
300 per min.

At the usual paper speed of 25 mm. per second (five large boxes), when the heart rate is *300 beats per minute,* the interval is *one large box (5 mm., 0.2 sec.) between two QRS complexes.* All that is necessary to determine heart rate when the rhythm is regular is to count the number of large boxes between two QRS complexes and divide into 300.

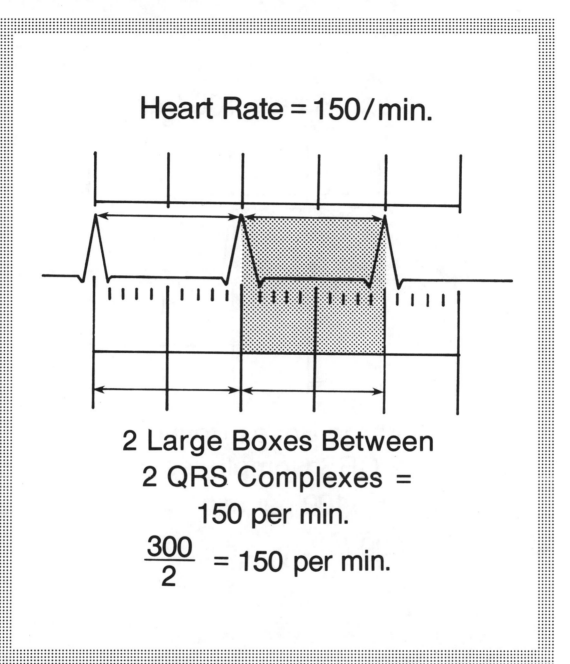

When the heart rate is 150 beats per minute, the interval is *two large boxes (0.4 sec.) between two QRS complexes (300/2)*. This determination is facilitated if you start the count with a QRS complex or P wave, whichever you are measuring, that falls on a heavy line.

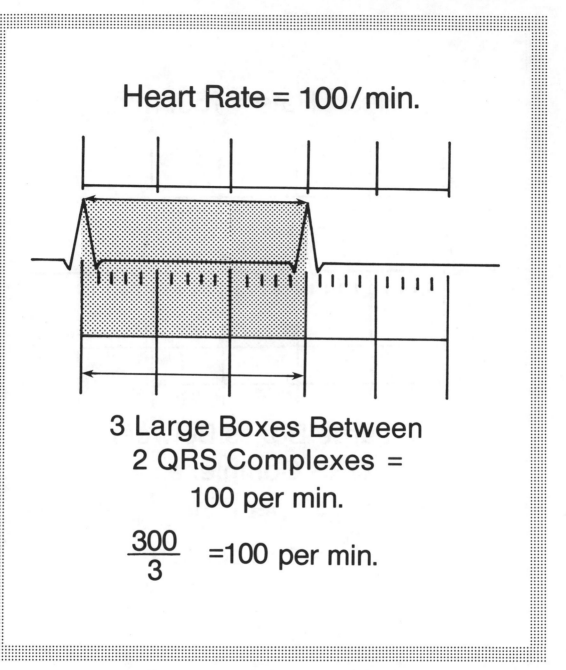

Heart Rate = 100/min.

**3 Large Boxes Between
2 QRS Complexes =
100 per min.**

$$\frac{300}{3} = 100 \text{ per min.}$$

When the heart is 100 per minute, the interval is *three large boxes (0.6 sec.) between two QRS complexes (300/3)*. This method permits a rapid determination of heart rate when the rhythm is regular.

Determination of Heart Rate Summary

Interval (No. of Large Boxes) Between 2 QRS Complexes	Rate/min.
1	300 (300÷1)
2	150 (300÷2)
3	100 (300÷3)
4	75 (300÷4)
5	60 (300÷5)
6	50 (300÷6)
7	43 (300÷7)
8	38 (300÷8)
9	33 (300÷9)
10	30 (300÷10)

This relationship permits the determination of heart rate using only two QRS complexes when the rhythm is regular. Simply count the number of large boxes and any fraction, and divide into 300 for the heart rate. When the rhythm is irregular, you have to count numerous QRS complexes to arrive at the proper average.

Practice
Determination of Heart Rate

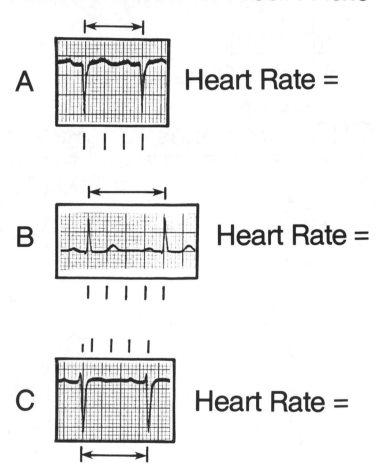

A   Heart Rate =

B   Heart Rate =

C   Heart Rate =

Answers:

A. Three large boxes between two QRS complexes: heart rate = 100 per minute (300 ÷ 3 = 100).

B. Four large boxes between two QRS complexes: heart rate = 75 per minute (300 ÷ 4 = 75).

C. Three and a half large boxes between two QRS complexes: heart rate = 86 per minute (300 ÷ 3.5 = 86).

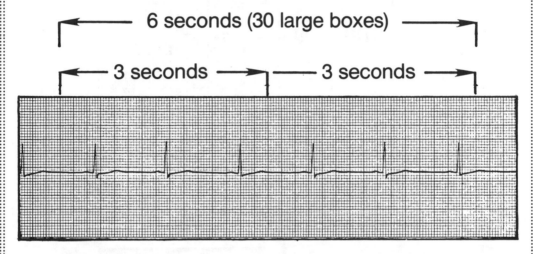

Heart Rate Determination
Another Method

6 seconds (30 large boxes)

3 seconds — 3 seconds

QRS Complexes in 6 sec. x 10 = Heart Rate

Another method of determining heart rate is to utilize the 3-second markers (15 large boxes = 3 seconds) at the upper border of the electrocardiographic paper. Count the number of QRS complexes in a six-second period and multiply by 10 for the rate per minute. Within the 6-second period above there are six QRS complexes. Therefore, the heart rate is 6 × 10 = 60 beats per minute. This method is especially useful when the rhythm is not regular.

Very often the electrocardiographic paper has been cut down so that the marks are not evident. In that case, count 30 large boxes and the number of QRS complexes within the 30 boxes and multiply by 10.

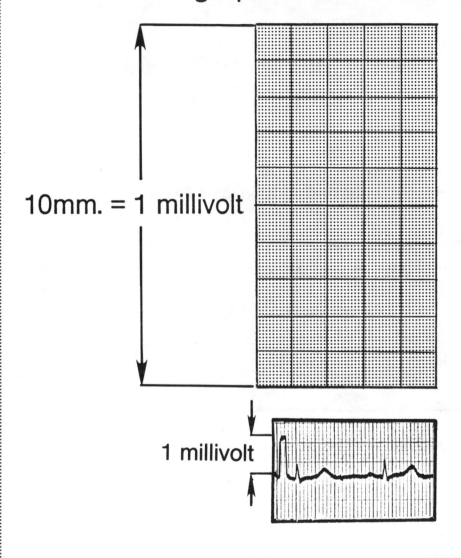

Electrocardiographic Standardization

10mm. = 1 millivolt

1 millivolt

The usual standardization on the electrocardiogram of 1 millivolt results in a deflection of two large boxes (10 mm.). The standardization is essential in order to properly evaluate the size of the deflections.

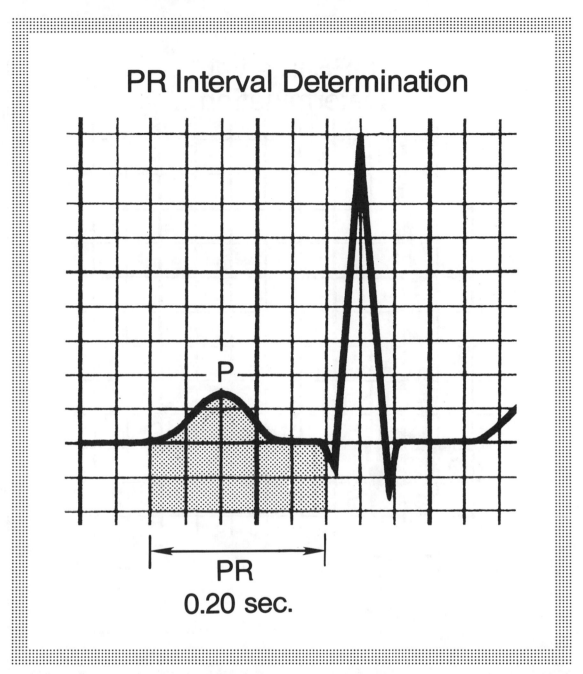

PR Interval Determination

The PR interval (from the beginning of the P wave to the beginning of the QRS complex) is 0.20 sec. (five small boxes or one large box). *The normal PR interval is from 0.12 to 0.20 sec.* This is an important measurement, since an abnormal prolongation represents a problem in the transmission of the electrical impulse from the atria to the ventricles.

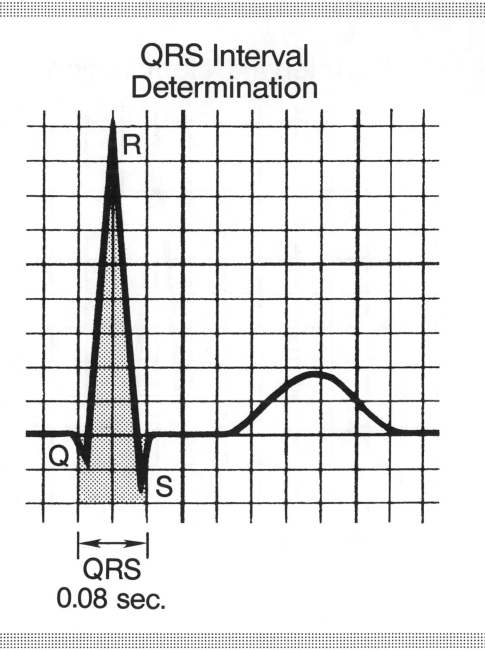

QRS Interval Determination

QRS 0.08 sec.

The QRS interval (QRS complex duration) is 0.08 sec. (two small boxes). *The normal interval for ventricular depolarization* is up to 0.1 sec. (two and a half small boxes). This measurement is important because a normal QRS interval is found in rhythms originating above the ventricles (sinus, atrial and junctional). These rhythms will be studied shortly.

Practice

Determine the PR and QRS Intervals

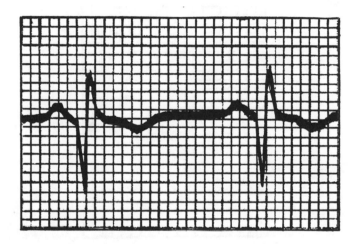

Answers:

The PR interval is 0.14 (3.5 × 0.04) sec.
The QRS interval is 0.08 (2 × 0.04) sec.

Practice

Determine the PR and QRS Intervals

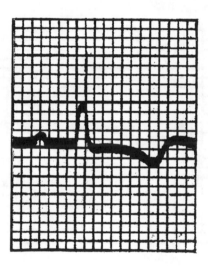

Answers:

The PR interval is 0.18 (4.5 × 0.04) sec.
The QRS interval is 0.06 (1.5 × 0.04) sec.

Practice

Determine the PR and QRS Intervals

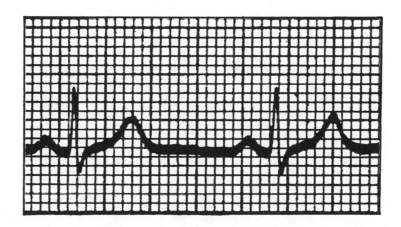

Answers:

The PR interval is 0.16 (4 × 0.04) sec.
The QRS interval is 0.08 (2 × 0.04) sec.

Chapter 3

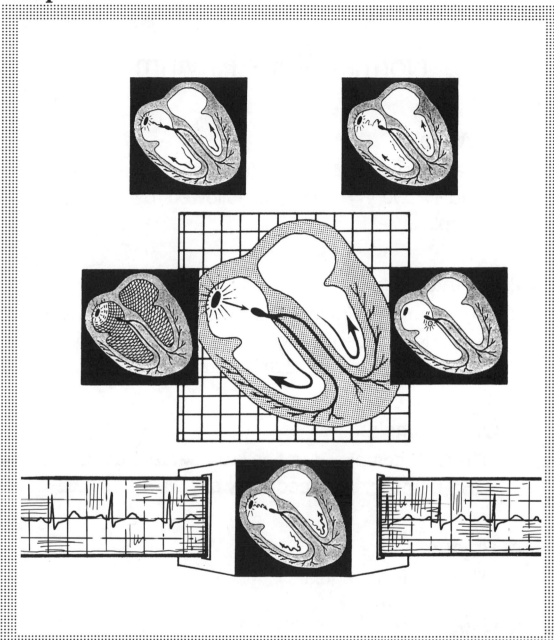

Normal Sinus Rhythm and Sinus Rhythm Alterations

Normal Sinus Rhythm

Sinus Tachycardia

Sinus Bradycardia

Sinus Arrhythmia

Sinus Arrest

Sinoatrial (SA) Block

Normal Sinus Rhythm

1. P Wave:

The P waves are positive (upright) and uniform in lead II. Every P wave is followed by a QRS complex.

2. PR Interval:

The normal PR interval (from the beginning of the P wave to the beginning of the QRS complex) is constant between 0.12 and 0.2 sec.

3. QRS Complex:

The QRS complex duration is 0.1 sec. or less. Every QRS complex is preceded by a P wave.

4. Rhythm:

The rhythm is regular.

5. Rate:

The rate is between 60 and 100 per minute. It is quite constant at a given rate, varying less than 10%.

Normal Sinus Rhythm

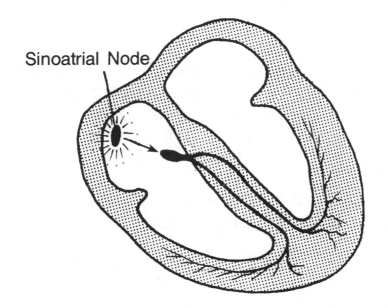

Sinoatrial Node

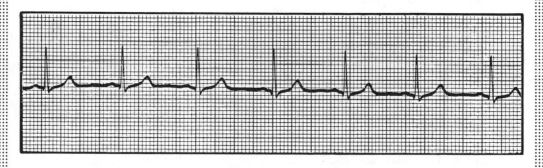

In order to describe the rhythm of the heart as *normal sinus rhythm* (the impulse originating in the sinoatrial [SA] node, the normal pacemaker of the heart) without qualifications, the indicated criteria must be met.

In addition to the sinus rhythms and sinus rhythm alterations, we will be studying atrial, junctional and ventricular arrhythmias as well as atrioventricular (AV) conduction disturbances. Every abnormality will vary in some respect from normal sinus rhythm. Any beat or rhythm originating outside the *SA node* is an *ectopic* beat or rhythm, ectopic in that it does not originate in the normal site.

Sinus Tachycardia

1. P Wave:

The P waves are positive and uniform in lead II. Every P wave is followed by a QRS complex.

2. PR Interval:

The PR interval is normal between 0.12 and 0.2 sec. and is constant from beat to beat.

3. QRS Complex:

The QRS complex duration is 0.1 sec. or less. Every QRS complex is preceded by a P wave.

4. Rhythm:

The rhythm is regular.

5. Rate:

The rate is constant above 100 (100-160) per minute.

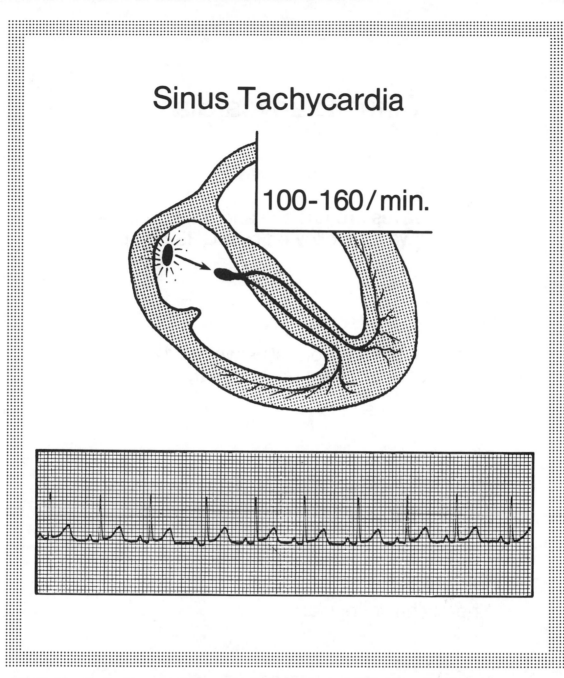

If all the criteria for normal sinus rhythm have been fulfilled but the heart rate is greater than 100 beats per minute, the rhythm is called *sinus tachycardia*. Tachycardia means fast heart. The range for sinus tachycardia is 100 to 160 beats per minute. The word sinus appearing before the tachycardia indicates that the origin of the rhythm is the SA node, the normal pacemaker of the heart.

Sinus Bradycardia

1. P Wave:

The P waves are positive and uniform in lead II. Every P wave is followed by a QRS complex.

2. PR Interval:

The PR interval is normal between 0.12 and 0.2 sec. and is constant from beat to beat.

3. QRS Complex:

The QRS complex duration is 0.1 sec. or less. Every QRS complex is preceded by a P wave.

4. Rhythm:

The rhythm is regular.

5. Rate:

The rate is constant below 60 per minute.

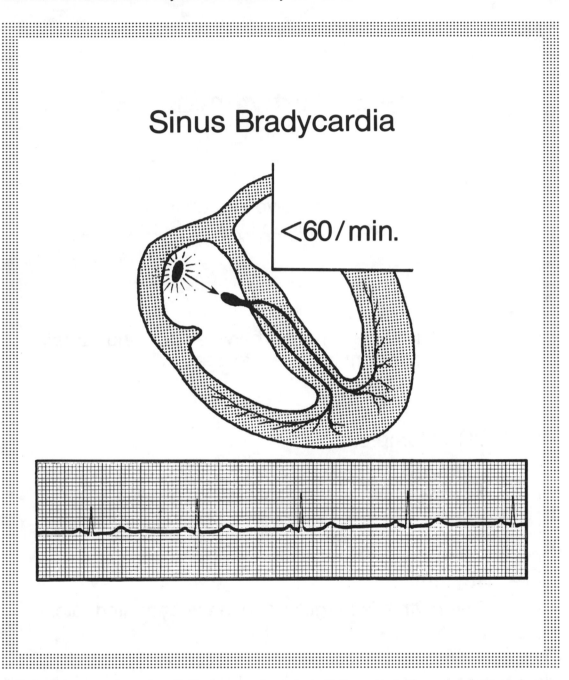

Sinus Bradycardia

<60/min.

If the heart rate is under 60 beats per minute but all the criteria for normal sinus rhythm have been fulfilled, the rhythm is known as *sinus bradycardia*. Bradycardia means slow heart.

Sinus Arrhythmia

1. P Wave:

The P waves are positive and uniform in lead II. Every P wave is followed by a QRS complex.

2. PR Interval:

The PR interval is normal between 0.12 and 0.2 sec. and is constant from beat to beat.

3. QRS Complex:

The QRS complex duration is 0.1 sec. or less. Every QRS complex is preceded by a P wave.

4. Rhythm:

The rhythm is irregular due to the changing rate.

5. Rate:

The rate varies by more than 10%.

Sinus Arrhythmia

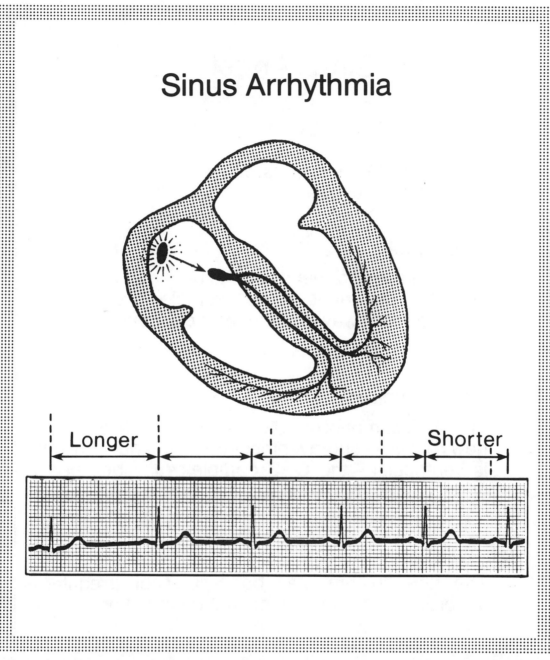

Sinus arrhythmia meets all the criteria described under normal sinus rhythm except for the variation in rate, often associated with the respiratory cycles. It is commonly seen in young people. The PR intervals are constant, but the RR intervals are continually changing. The heart rate in this electrocardiogram varies from 53 to 68 beats per minute, more than 10%.

Sinus Arrest

1. P Wave:

Since the SA node has ceased functioning, no "sinus" P waves are visible.

2. PR Interval:

The PR interval depends on the pacemaker that becomes dominant. In the example given (p.51) there are no P waves after the arrest, hence no PR interval.

3. QRS Complex:

The QRS complex duration is 0.1 sec. or less if the new rhythm is supraventricular [1]. If the new rhythm is ventricular [2] the QRS complex may be very wide, greater than 0.12 sec. and bizarre.

4. Rhythm:

The new rhythm may be regular or irregular according to the new dominant pacemaker.

5. Rate:

The rate will vary according to the new rhythm.

[1,2] See p. 51.

Sinus Arrest

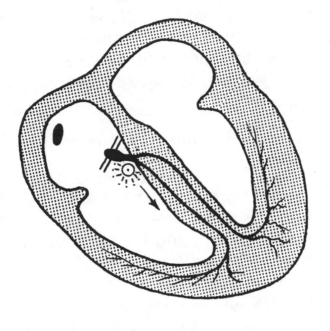

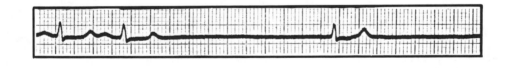

Sinus arrest is a sudden failure of the SA node to initiate an expected impulse. Fortunately, a lower pacemaker often becomes dominant, initiating a new rhythm (in this case, AV junctional— to be described shortly).

---

[1] The supraventricular rhythms, in addition to normal sinus rhythm, are the atrial and AV junctional rhythms. These will be studied in Chapters 4 and 5.

[2] The characteristic QRS complex of ventricular origin is wide and bizarre. This will be studied in Chapter 6.

Sinoatrial (SA) Block

1. P Wave:

The P waves are positive and uniform in lead II. However, an entire cycle (P, QRS and T) is missing. The SA node initiates an impulse, but it is not propagated to the atria; it is blocked and hence there is no P wave. The pause is a multiple of the regular cycle length.

2. PR Interval:

The PR interval is normal between 0.12 and 0.2 sec. and is constant from beat to beat except during the pause when an entire cycle is missing. Also, the PR interval may be slightly shorter following the pause, as illustrated in the example on p. 53.

3. QRS Complex:

The QRS complex duration is 0.1 sec. or less except during the pause, when an entire cycle is missing.

4. Rhythm:

The rhythm may be regular or irregular, according to the number and position of the missing cycles.

5. Rate:

The rate may be constant or varying, according to the number and position of the missing cycles.

Sinoatrial (SA) Block

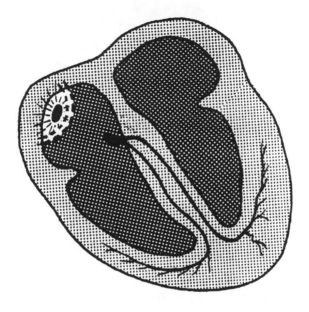

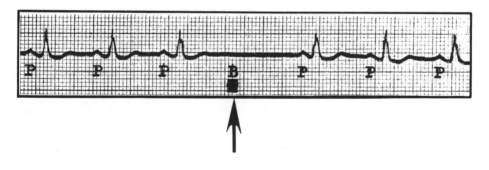

In *sinoatrial (SA) block,* the SA node initiates the impulse but the *propagation* is blocked, so that the atria are not depolarized and, therefore, there is no P wave. SA block represents a failure of impulse propagation rather than of impulse formation. The pause is a multiple of the regular cycle length. The block, represented by the letter B above (arrow), is seen where the P should normally be.

Rhythm Analysis

1. P Wave:

2. PR Interval:

3. QRS Complex:

4. Rhythm:

5. Rate:

Impression and Comment:

Utilizing all the information studied so far, we can analyze arrhythmias following the five steps enumerated above.

Practice
Rhythm Analysis

Practice
Rhythm Analysis

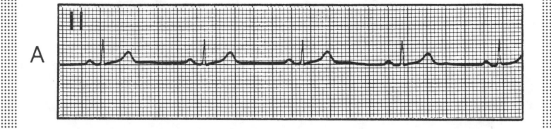

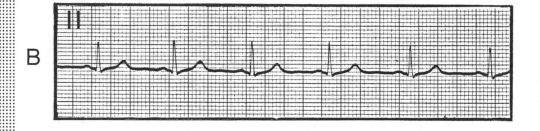

Analysis A: **Analysis B:**

RHYTHM ANALYSIS

A. 1. P Wave:
    The P waves are positive and uniform in lead II. Every P wave is followed by a QRS complex.
    2. PR Interval:
    The PR interval is 0.16 sec.
    3. QRS Complex:
    The QRS complex duration is 0.08 sec. Every QRS complex is preceded by a P wave.
    4. Rhythm:
    The rhythm is regular.
    5. Rate:
    The rate is 57 beats per minute.

Impression and Comment:

Sinus Bradycardia. All the criteria for normal sinus rhythm have been met except for rate, which is below 60 beats per minute.

B. 1. P Wave:
    The P waves are positive and uniform in lead II. Every P wave is followed by a QRS complex.
    2. PR Interval:
    The PR interval is constant at 0.16 sec.
    3. QRS Complex:
    The QRS complex duration is 0.08 sec. Every QRS complex is preceded by a P wave.
    4. Rhythm:
    The rhythm is regular.
    5. Rate:
    The rate is 73 beats per minute.

Impression and Comment:

Normal sinus rhythm. The slight variation in heart rate (71 to 75 beats per minute, less than 10%) does not interfere with the diagnosis of normal sinus rhythm.

Chapter 4

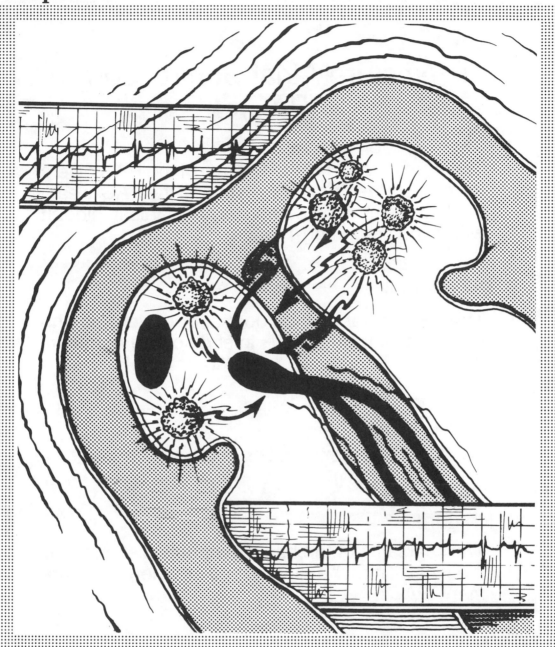

Atrial Arrhythmias

Premature Atrial Contraction
(PAC)
Premature Atrial Contraction
(Blocked)

Atrial Tachycardia
Atrial Flutter
Atrial Fibrillation
Multifocal Atrial Tachycardia

Premature Atrial Contraction (PAC)

1. P Wave:

The configuration of the P wave of the PAC differs from that of the dominant rhythm. If the PAC is early, the P wave may be completely or partially hidden within the preceding T wave.

2. PR Interval:

The PR interval may be normal or prolonged and often differs from the PR interval of the dominant rhythm.

3. QRS Complex:

The QRS complex duration is 0.1 sec. or less.

4. Rhythm:

The regularity of the basic rhythm is disturbed by the PAC. It may be quite irregular when there are many PACs.

5. Rate:

The rate depends on the basic rhythm and the number of PACs present.

Premature Atrial Contraction (PAC)

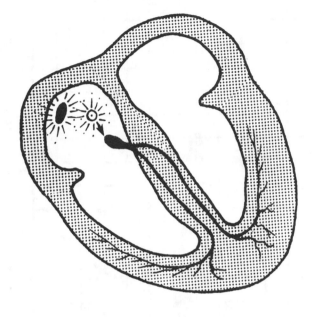

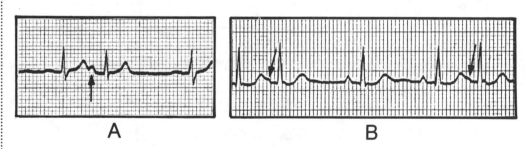

A   B

Premature contractions (PACs) of the atria are seen when an *ectopic atrial pacemaker* propagates an impulse before the next normal beat is due. The PACs may be conducted to the ventricles, as seen above. The P wave of the PAC differs from the sinus P wave in contour. In general, following PACs, the PR interval may be normal or prolonged, and the QRS complex may be of normal contour and duration or of changed configuration and prolonged, depending on the state of refractoriness of the conduction tissue. Also, the PACs may herald paroxysms of atrial tachycardia. Note that the P waves (arrows) of the PACs in (A) and (B) are partially hidden within the preceding T waves. The earlier P waves in (B) are more completely hidden.

Refractory Periods

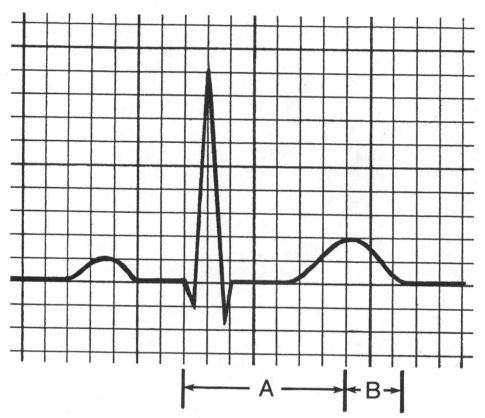

|←———— A ————→|←B→|

A. Absolute Refractory Period
B. Relative Refractory Period

In order to understand why a PAC is blocked (not conducted), it is important to know when the absolute and relative refractory periods of the ventricle occur. Earlier (pp. 3–4), the processes of depolarization and repolarization were described. The process of depolarization reflects the flow of an electrical current to all cells along the pathway of conduction. The cells then return to their original resting state by the process of repolarization. Ventricular repolarization is complete at the end of the T wave (pp. 14–15), permitting a new impulse to start the process again.

A new impulse, occurring before the peak of the T wave, finds the ventricular conduction system unable to accept it. This is the *absolute refractory period*. Although the downslope of the T

Premature Atrial Contractions

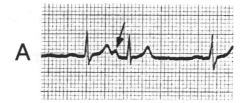

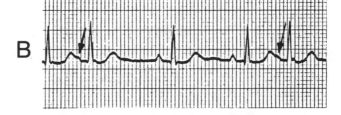

PAC Blocked

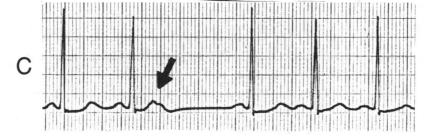

wave is still within the refractory period, an impulse may be conducted under certain circumstances. This is the *relative refractory period.* Note that the PACs in (A) and (B) occur during the relative refractory period and are followed by QRS complexes. In (C), the PAC occurs during the absolute refractory period and is not followed by ventricular depolarization (QRS complex). The PAC is blocked, not conducted.

Atrial Tachycardia

1. P Wave:

The P wave differs in configuration from the sinus P wave. It may, however, be hidden in the preceding T wave and not be seen as a separate entity due to the rapid rate.

2. PR Interval:

The PR interval is between 0.12 and 0.2 sec. and is constant from beat to beat. The PR interval may not be measurable if the P wave is partially or completely hidden in the preceding T wave.

3. QRS Complex:

The QRS complex duration is 0.1 sec. or less. Every QRS complex is preceded by a P wave.

4. Rhythm:

The rhythm is regular.

5. Rate:

The rate is constant between 160 and 250 per minute.

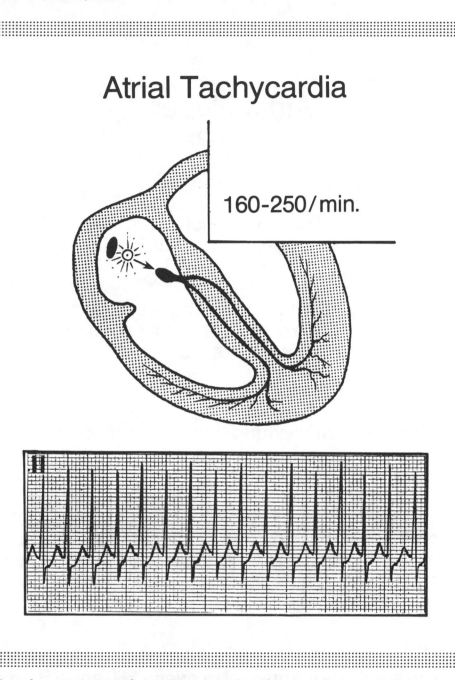

Atrial Tachycardia

160-250/min.

The SA node can emit impulses up to approximately 160 per minute in the resting state. If the rate is above 160, another pacemaker must be considered. Here the SA node is no longer the dominant pacemaker at a rate of 240 per minute. *Atrial tachycardia* is characterized by a rapid (160 to 250 beats per minute) rate and regular rhythm, sudden in onset, often terminating abruptly; it may be followed by a pause. The P waves, when seen, differ from the sinus P waves in contour.

Atrial Flutter

1. P Wave (F Wave):

The atrial deflections, which often have a "saw-tooth" appearance, are known as F or flutter waves.

2. PR Interval:

Because of the characteristic appearance of the flutter waves, it is often difficult to determine the PR interval. It is therefore, not measured.

3. QRS Complex:

The QRS complex duration is 0.1 sec. or less.

4. Rhythm:

The rhythm may be regular or irregular, depending on the relationship of atrial to ventricular beats. In the example given (p. 67), the rhythm is regular with a 4:1 conduction ratio (four atrial beats for every ventricular beat).

5. Rate:

The atrial rate is constant between 250 and 350 per minute. The ventricular rate depends on the conduction ratio between the atria and ventricles.

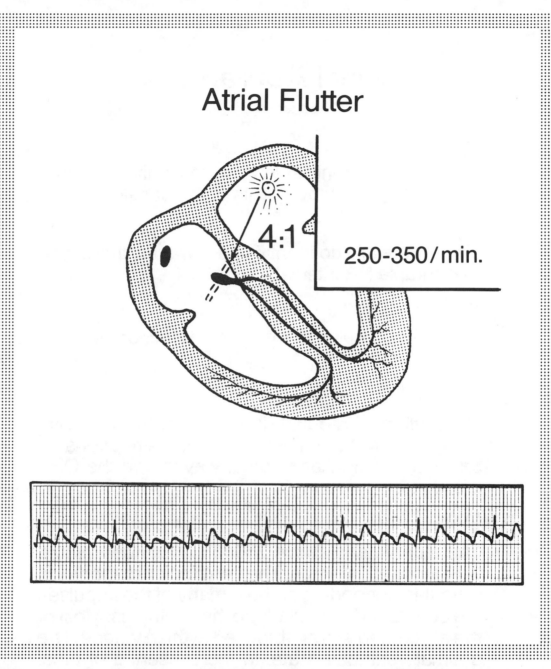

Atrial Flutter

4:1

250-350/min.

The *fluttering atria* are represented by the undulating waves, rising and falling to the baseline. Note the saw-tooth character of the atrial waves (F or flutter waves). The atrial rate is 300 beats per minute, whereas the ventricular rate is 75 beats per minute, with a ratio of 4:1. The atrial rate in atrial flutter is usually 250 to 350 beats per minute. The AV node protects the ventricles by not allowing every impulse that reaches it to be transmitted to the ventricles. Only one of four impulses is reaching the ventricles, as illustrated; hence there is 4:1 atrioventricular conduction.

Atrial Fibrillation

1. P Wave:

There are no identifiable P waves, only fibrillatory waves, irregular movements of the baseline.

2. PR Interval:

Since there are no identifiable P waves, there is no measurable PR interval.

3. QRS Complex:

The QRS complex duration is 0.1 sec. or less.

4. Rhythm:

The rhythm is irregularly irregular, i.e. irregular with no specific pattern. There is no stable relationship between the fibrillatory atrial waves and the QRS complexes.

5. Rate:

The atrial rate is above 350 (350-600) per minute with a chaotic rhythm. The ventricular response is irregular, depending on how many of the impulses are conducted, irregularly, to the ventricles. Most of the atrial impulses are blocked at the AV node. The optimal ventricular rate, in the presence of atrial fibrillation, is between 60 and 100 per minute. If it is below 60 it is considered a slow ventricular response; if it is over 100 it is considered a rapid ventricular response.

Atrial Fibrillation

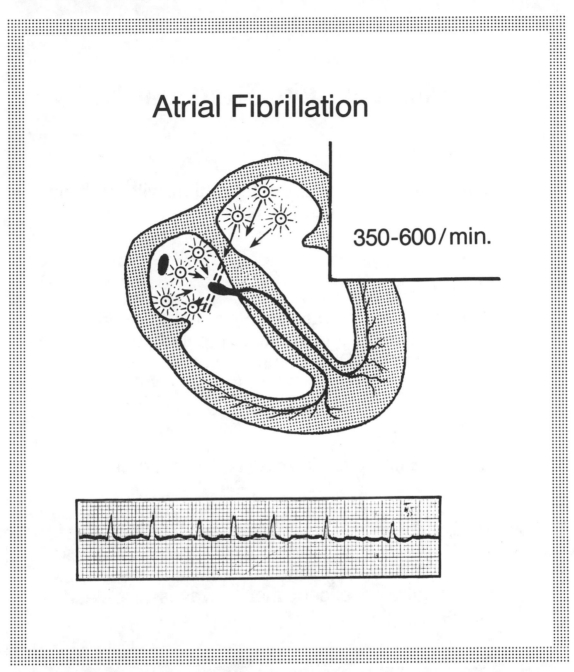

350-600/min.

    Disorganized, ineffective contractions of the atria (350 to 600 beats per minute) characterize *atrial fibrillation.* No P waves are seen, and the ventricular response is irregular, depending on how many of the 350 to 600 impulses are conducted to the ventricles. If the atrial rate is 500 beats per minute and the ventricular rate is 125 beats per minute, it means that one in four atrial impulses is conducted, irregularly, to the ventricles. This rhythm has been described as irregularly irregular.

Multifocal Atrial Tachycardia

1. P Wave:

The P waves vary in configuration, with multiple atrial foci initiating impulses.

2. PR Interval:

The PR intervals vary from normal to prolonged. There is no stable relationship between the P waves and the QRS complexes.

3. QRS Complex:

The QRS complex duration is 0.1 sec. or less.

4. Rhythm:

The rhythm is irregularly irregular and resembles atrial fibrillation except that P waves are clearly visible.

5. Rate:

The rate is not constant from beat to beat because of multiple atrial foci, often above 170 per minute.

Multifocal Atrial Tachycardia

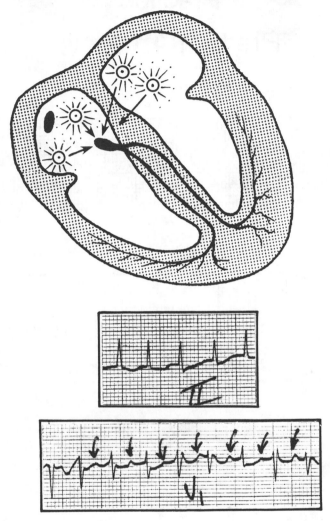

Multifocal (chaotic) atrial tachycardia is sometimes mistaken for atrial fibrillation, since the rhythm is also irregularly irregular. At a quick glance, lead II might appear to be an example of atrial fibrillation. Lead V_1, analogous to the monitoring lead MCL_1 (see p. 25), however, reveals the different P wave contours as well as the varying PR intervals. This rhythm is frequently found in patients with chronic obstructive pulmonary disease associated with hypoxia.

Practice
Rhythm Analysis

A
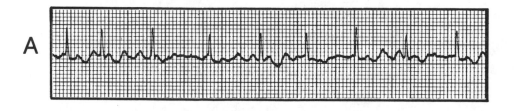

B
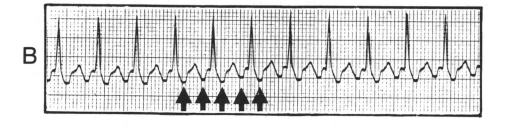

Analysis A: **Analysis B:**

RHYTHM ANALYSIS

A. 1. P Wave:
        There are no identifiable P waves, only fibrillatory waves, irregular movements of the baseline.
    2. PR Interval:
        Since there are no identifiable P waves, there is no measurable PR interval.
    3. QRS Complex:
        The QRS complex duration is 0.04 sec.
    4. Rhythm:
        The rhythm is irregularly irregular.
    5. Rate:
        The atrial rate is above 350 beats per minute, with a chaotic rhythm. The ventricular response is irregular with an average rate of 120 beats per minute.

Impression and Comment:

Atrial Fibrillation with a rapid ventricular response of 120 beats per minute. There is no stable relationship between the fibrillatory atrial waves and the QRS complexes. Most of the atrial impulses are blocked at the AV node.

B. 1   P Wave:
        The atrial deflections, often with a saw-tooth appearance, are known as flutter waves.
    2. PR Interval:
        Due to the characteristic appearance of the flutter waves, it is often difficult to determine the PR interval. It is, therefore, not measured.
    3. QRS Complex:
        The QRS complex duration is 0.06 sec.
    4. Rhythm:
        The rhythm is regular with a 2:1 conduction ratio (two atrial beats for every ventricular beat).
    5. Rate:
        The atrial rate is 300 and the ventricular rate is 150 beats per minute.

Impression and Comment:

Atrial Flutter with a 2:1 conduction ratio. The AV node is protecting the heart by permitting only one of two atrial impulses to be transmitted to the ventricles. The arrows point to some of the flutter waves.

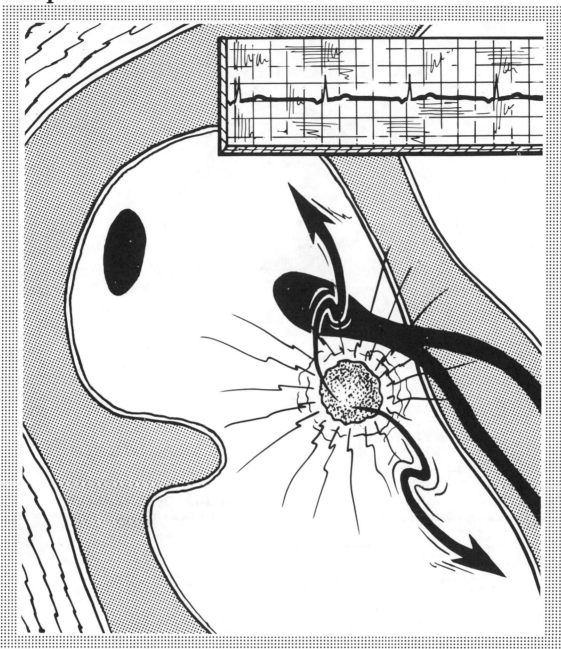

Chapter 5

Junctional Arrhythmias

Junctional Rhythm
Premature Junctional Contraction
(PJC)
Junctional Escape Rhythm

Junctional Tachycardia
Accelerated Junctional Rhythm
Wandering Pacemaker
Supraventricular Tachycardia

Normal Sinus Rhythm

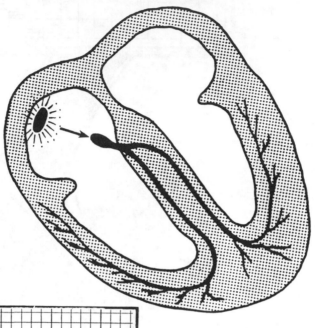

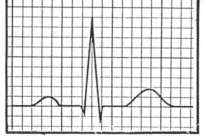

Normal Depolarization
of Atria

Normal Depolarization
of Ventricles

P Wave Positive (Upright) in Lead II

As was seen earlier, the normal pacemaker of the heart is the SA node. The electrical impulse, after the depolarization of the atria, spreads to the AV node and bundle of His, to the left and right bundle branches and then to the Purkinje network with ventricular depolarization. This normal sequence of depolarization results in P waves that are *positive (upright)* in *lead II* (see p. 42).

The AV node, through which the impulses pass from the atria to the ventricles, is *not* a pacemaker. The pacemaker, which had once been thought to be in the AV node, is actually in the AV junction (junctional tissue between the atria and the ventricles).

Junctional Rhythm

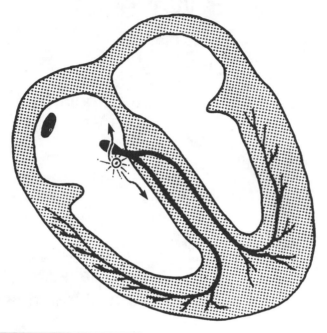

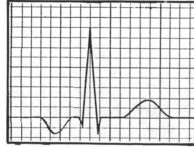

Retrograde Depolarization of Atria
Normal Depolarization of Ventricles

P Wave Negative (Inverted) in Lead II

When the AV junction becomes the dominant pacemaker, the single impulse originating in the AV junction spreads in *two* directions. The ventricles are depolarized normally, since the impulse spreads through the bundle of His to the bundle branches and then to the Purkinje network, leading to ventricular depolarization. The QRS complexes, therefore, are normal. The atria, however, are depolarized in a manner opposite to that of normal. This is known as *retrograde* atrial depolarization. This retrograde atrial depolarization is reflected electrocardiographically by a *negative* (downward, inverted) P wave in lead II.

Junctional Rhythm
P Waves

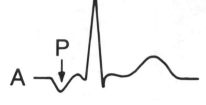

Atria Depolarized
Before Ventricles

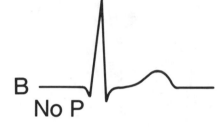

Simultaneous
Depolarization of
Atria and Ventricles

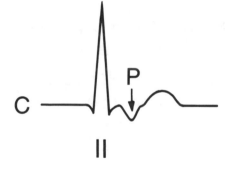

Ventricles Depolarized
Before Atria

The position of the P wave depends on whether

    A. The atria are depolarized *before* the ventricles. The P wave is inverted in lead II with a short (0.12 sec. or less) PR interval.

    B. The atria and ventricles are depolarized *simultaneously.* The P wave is then hidden within the QRS complex and is not visible on the electrocardiogram.

    C. The atria are depolarized *after* the ventricles. The P wave is then inverted in lead II, following the QRS complex.

An additional possibility exists, as illustrated on p. 79.

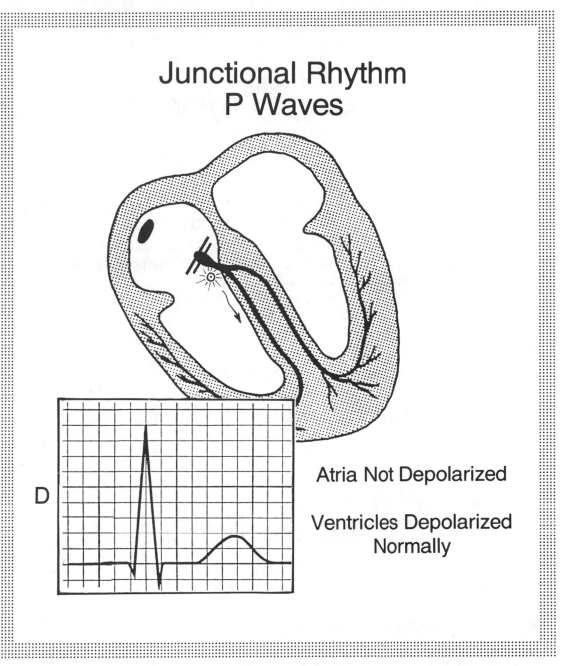

Junctional Rhythm
P Waves

Atria Not Depolarized

Ventricles Depolarized Normally

D. When no P waves are visible, a fourth possibility exists. The atria are not depolarized because retrograde conduction is blocked. The QRS complexes are normal, with normal ventricular depolarization.

Junctional Rhythm

1. P Wave:

When the P waves are present before or after the QRS complexes, they are inverted (negative) in lead II . Often no P waves are seen because they are either within the QRS complexes or there has been no atrial depolarization.

2. PR Interval:

When the inverted P waves are visible before the QRS complexes, the PR interval is short, 0.12 sec. or less. If the P waves are within or following the QRS complexes, no PR interval can be measured.

3. QRS Complex:

The QRS complex duration is 0.1 sec. or less.

4. Rhythm:

The rhythm is regular.

5. Rate:

The rate is constant between 40 and 60 per minute.

Junctional Rhythm

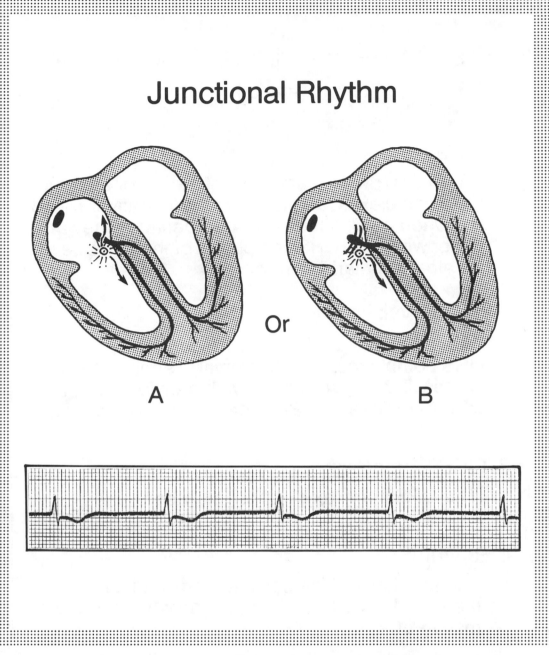

Or

A   B

When no P waves are present in junctional rhythm, two possibilities exist. Either the atria and ventricles are depolarized simultaneously (A), or there is retrograde block and the atria are not depolarized (B).

Premature Junctional Contraction (PJC)

1. P Wave:

When the P waves are present before or after the QRS complexes, they are inverted (negative) in lead ‖ . Often no P waves are seen because they are either within the QRS complexes or there has been no atrial depolarization.

2. PR Interval:

When the inverted P waves are visible before the QRS complexes, the PR interval is short, 0.12 sec. or less. If the P waves are within or following the QRS complexes, no PR interval can be measured.

3. QRS Complex:

The QRS complex duration is 0.1 sec. or less.

4. Rhythm:

The regularity of the basic rhythm is disturbed by the PJC. It may be quite irregular when there are many PJCs.

5. Rate:

The rate depends on the basic rhythm and the number of PJCs present.

Premature Junctional Contraction (PJC)

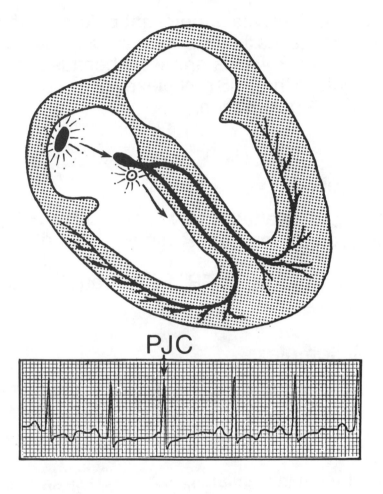

PJC

Premature junctional beats are seen when the AV junction propagates an impulse before the next normal beat is due. In the illustration above, the PJC is seen shortly after the onset of the sinus P wave and interrupts the sinus rhythm.

Junctional Escape Rhythm

1. P Wave:

   When the P waves are present before or after the QRS complexes they are inverted (negative) in lead II. Often no P waves are seen because they are either within the QRS complexes or there has been no atrial depolarization.

2. PR Interval:

   When the inverted P waves are visible before the QRS complexes, the PR interval is short, 0.12 sec. or less. If the P waves are within or following the QRS complexes, no PR interval can be measured.

3. QRS Complex:

   The QRS complex duration is 0.1 sec. or less.

4. Rhythm:

   The rhythm is regular.

5. Rate:

   The rate is that of the AV junctional pacemaker, 40-60 per minute, but it may vary.

Junctional Escape Rhythm

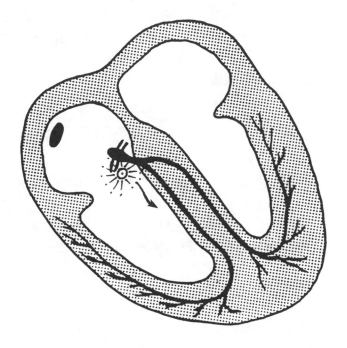

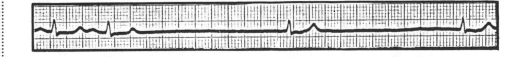

With the *arrest of the SA node* (see pp. 50–51), a long pause follows. The beat following this pause is known as an *escape* beat, usually from a lower pacemaker, often the AV junction, as above. If the pacemaker originating the escape beat remains the dominant one, the rhythm may then be called an *escape rhythm*.

Junctional Tachycardia

1. P Wave:

When the P waves are present before or after the QRS complexes, they are inverted (negative) in lead II. Often no P waves are seen because they are either within the QRS complexes or there has been no atrial depolarization.

2. PR Interval:

When the inverted P waves are visible before the QRS complexes, the PR interval is short, 0.12 sec. or less. If the P waves are within or following the QRS complexes, no PR interval can be measured.

3. QRS Complex:

The QRS complex duration is 0.1 sec. or less.

4. Rhythm:

The rhythm is regular.

5. Rate:

The rate is above 100 (100-170) per minute.

Junctional Tachycardia

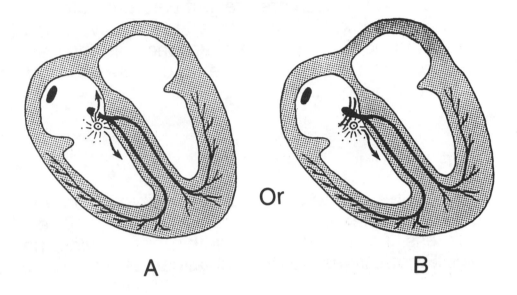

Or

A   B

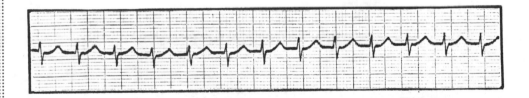

As seen earlier, when no P waves are present with a dominant junctional pacemaker, two possibilities exist. Either the atria and ventricles are depolarized simultaneously (A), or there is retrograde block and the atria are not depolarized (B).

Accelerated Junctional Rhythm

1. P Wave:

When the P waves are present before or after the QRS complexes, they are inverted (negative) in lead II. Often no P waves are seen because they are either within the QRS complexes or there has been no atrial depolarization.

2. PR Interval:

When the inverted P waves are visible before the QRS complexes, the PR interval is short, 0.12 sec. or less. If the P waves are within or following the QRS complexes, no PR interval can be measured.

3. QRS Complex:

The QRS complex duration is 0.1 sec. or less.

4. Rhythm:

The rhythm is regular.

5. Rate:

The rate is constant between 60 and 100 per minute.

Accelerated Junctional Rhythm

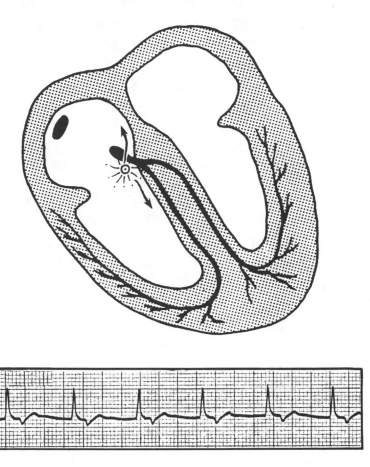

The inherent rate of the AV junctional pacemaker is 40 to 60 beats per minute. As seen on pp. 86–87, the rate is above 100 (100 to 170) beats per minute in junctional tachycardia. When the rate of the AV junction is between 60 and 100 (as above, at 88) beats per minute, the rhythm is known as an accelerated junctional rhythm. Note the inverted P waves following the QRS complexes.

Wandering Pacemaker

1. P Wave:

   The configuration of the P wave varies according to the pacemaker, since pacemaker dominance is shared by more than one pacemaker. In the example on page 91, the pacemaker shifts between the SA node with positive P waves and the AV junction with negative P waves.

2. PR Interval:

   The PR interval depends on the dominant pacemaker. The PR interval of the sinus beats is between 0.12 and 0.2 sec., and the PR interval of the junctional beats is 0.12 sec. or less and constant from beat to beat. In the example given, the PR interval is approximately 0.12 sec. for both the sinus and the junctional beats.

3. QRS Complex:

   The QRS complex duration is 0.1 sec. or less.

4. Rhythm:

   The rhythm may be slightly irregular with the shifting pacemaker sites.

5. Rate:

   The rate may vary with the shifting pacemaker sites.

Wandering Pacemaker

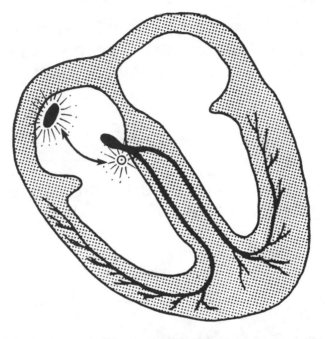

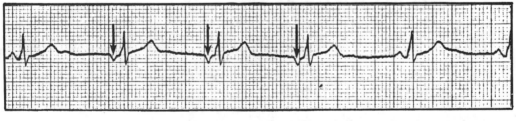

When pacemaker dominance is shared by more than one pacemaker, P waves of varying configurations result. This is known as a *wandering pacemaker.* Here pacemaker dominance is shared by the SA node and the AV junction. Notice the variation in P wave polarity. Following a sinus beat, there are three junctional beats (arrows) followed by two sinus beats.

Supraventricular Tachycardia

1. P Wave:

   P waves, because of the rate (188 in the example given on page 93), cannot be clearly delineated to establish the diagnosis as atrial or junctional.

2. PR Interval:

   No P waves are seen; therefore, there is no measurable PR interval.

3. QRS Complex:

   The QRS complex duration is 0.1 sec. or less.

4. Rhythm:

   The rhythm is regular.

5. Rate:

   The rate is generally above 150 per minute.

Supraventricular Tachycardia

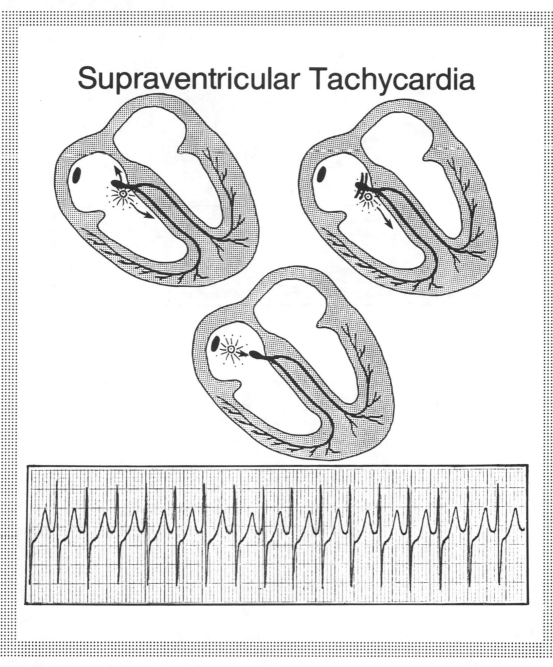

Often the P waves, because of the rate (188 above), cannot be clearly delineated to establish the diagnosis as atrial or junctional tachycardia. Such a tachycardia is frequently classified under the overall category of *supraventricular tachycardia,* originating *above* the ventricles. The normal QRS interval (0.1 sec. or less) identifies a supraventricular pacemaker.

Practice
Rhythm Analysis

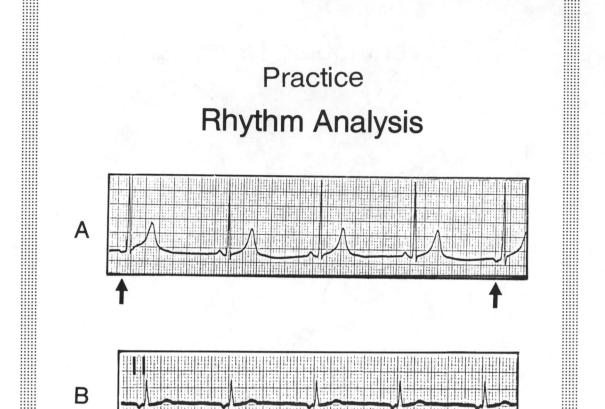

Analysis A: **Analysis B:**

RHYTHM ANALYSIS

A. 1. P Wave:
        The first and fifth P waves are negative (arrows), whereas the second, third and fourth
        are positive.
    2. PR Interval:
        Where the P waves are negative, the PR interval is 0.12 sec., and where the P waves
        are positive, the PR interval is 0.16 sec.
    3. QRS Complex:
        The QRS complex duration is 0.07 sec.
    4. Rhythm:
        The rhythm is slightly irregular with the shifting pacemaker sites.
    5. Rate:
        The rate varies from 41 to 48 beats per minute (average is 45 beats per minute) with
        the shifting pacemaker sites.

Impression and Comment:

Wandering Pacemaker. The pacemaker is wandering between the SA node and AV junction.

B. 1. P Wave:
        The P waves preceding the QRS complexes are inverted in lead II.
    2. PR Interval:
        The PR interval is 0.08 sec.
    3. QRS Complex:
        The QRS complex duration is 0.06 sec.
    4. Rhythm:
        The rhythm is regular.
    5. Rate:
        The rate is 60 beats per minute.

Impression and Comment:

Junctional Rhythm. The intrinsic rate of the junctional pacemaker is 40 to 60 beats per minute.

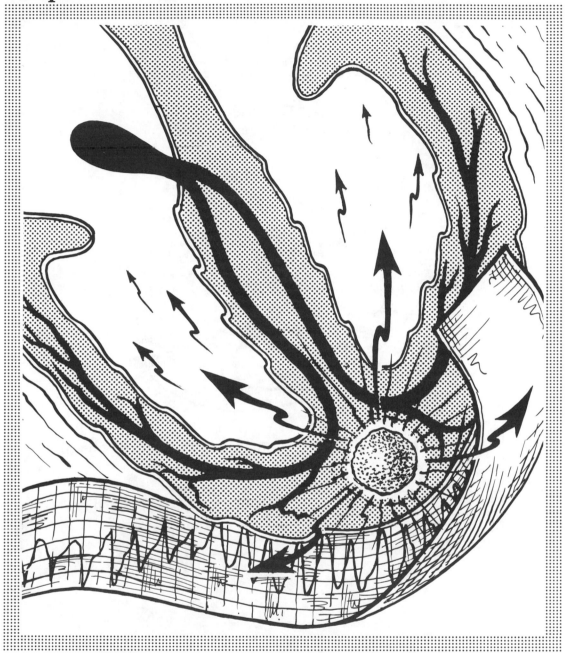

Chapter 6

Ventricular Arrhythmias

Idioventricular Rhythm
Premature Ventricular Contraction
(PVC)
Ventricular Tachycardia

Accelerated Idioventricular Rhythm
(AIVR)
Ventricular Flutter
Ventricular Fibrillation

Normal Sinus Rhythm

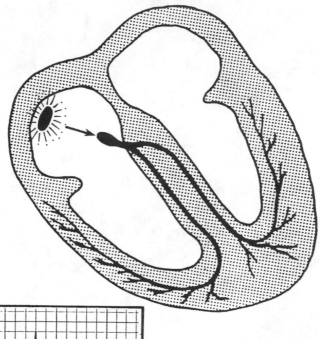

Normal Depolarization
of Atria

Normal Depolarization
of Ventricles

QRS Interval-Up to
0.1 sec.

Until now, we have been studying arrhythmias originating in the SA node, atria and AV junction. These are supraventricular foci, with the pacemaker above the ventricles. Common to the supraventricular arrhythmias is a QRS complex that is normal in duration. The QRS complex duration is 0.1 sec. (two and a half small boxes) or less. Exceptions to this are explained on pp. 122–125. In order to have a QRS complex duration of 0.1 sec. or less, the normal pathways of conduction, specialized for rapid conduction, are used. An impulse

Ventricular Rhythm

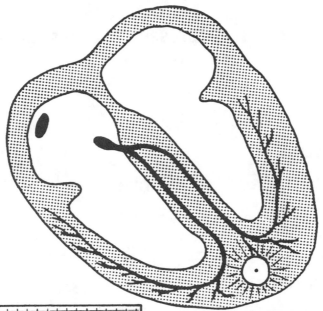

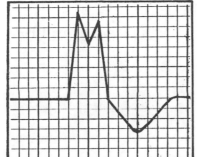

Abnormal Depolarization of Ventricles

Atria May or May Not Be Depolarized Retrogradely

QRS Interval Wide, Greater Than 0.1 sec.

originating in the *ventricles* follows an abnormal pathway of conduction and cannot depolarize the ventricles within 0.1 sec. or less. In a ventricular rhythm the QRS complex is, therefore, abnormally wide, greater than 0.1 sec., and frequently greater than 0.12 sec. (three small boxes). The QRS complex is not only wide but also often bizarre in appearance. The T wave is generally opposite the QRS in orientation. Above we have a positive QRS complex, wide and bizarre, with a negative T wave.

Idioventricular Rhythm

1. P Wave:

P waves may not be present, as illustrated on p. 101.

2. PR Interval:

There is no measurable PR interval.

3. QRS Complex:

The QRS complex duration is wide, greater than 0.1 sec., often greater than 0.12 sec. (three small boxes).

4. Rhythm:

The rhythm is regular.

5. Rate:

The rate is that of the ventricular pacemaker, 20 to 40 per minute.

Idioventricular Rhythm

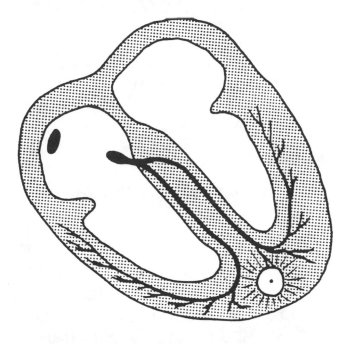

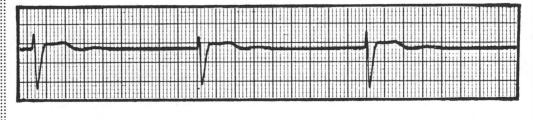

The inherent rate of the ventricular pacemaker is 20 to 40 beats per minute. The above rate is 33 per minute. With abnormal ventricular depolarization, the ventricular pacemaker is not as efficient as the supraventricular pacemakers. It is the lowest of the series of pacemakers and may become dominant when the higher pacemakers have failed. It may be an "escape" or "safety" rhythm and should not be suppressed.

Premature Ventricular Contraction (PVC)

1. P Wave:

The premature ventricular deflection (QRS complex) is not proceeded by a P wave.

2. PR Interval:

There is no measurable PR interval.

3. QRS Complex:

The QRS complex duration is at least 0.12 sec. The QRS complex is often bizarre in appearance compared with the normal QRS complexes.

4. Rhythm:

The regularity of the basic rhythm is disturbed by the PVC. It may be quite irregular when there are many PVCs.

5. Rate:

The rate depends on the basic rhythm and the number of PVCs present.

Premature Ventricular Contraction (PVC)

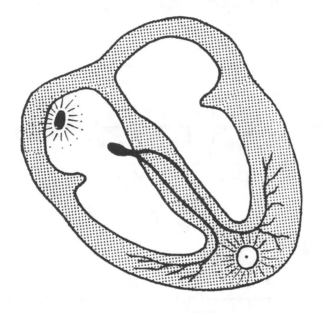

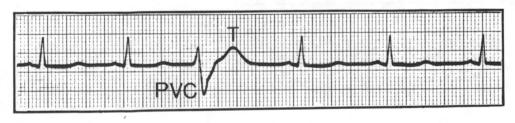

PVC

A *premature ventricular contraction* (PVC) is seen when an impulse is propagated from a ventricular focus before the next normal beat is due. The QRS complex is commonly widened and not preceded by a P wave. There may be retrograde activation of the atria following a premature contraction, or the normal sinus P waves may continue. Note that the T wave of the PVC is opposite the QRS complex in direction.

Premature Ventricular Contractions
Full Compensatory Pause

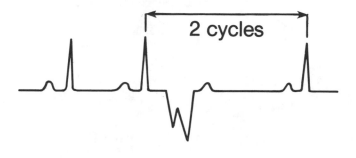

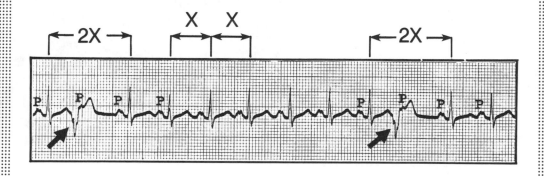

A PVC is frequently identified by the accompanying *compensatory pause*. The interval between the QRS complex before the PVC and the complex following the PVC is twice that of the regular cycle interval. This occurs because the PVC does not interfere with the pacemaking activity of the SA node. The sinus P waves following the PVCs are blocked, however, because they occur during the absolute refractory period (see pp. 62 and 63).

Premature Ventricular Contraction
Partial Compensatory Pause

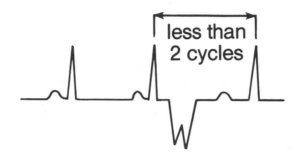

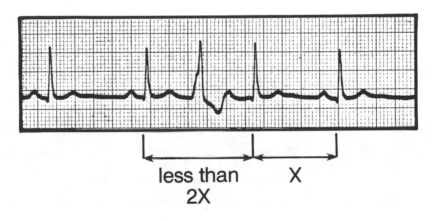

At times the interval between the QRS complex before the PVC and the complex following the PVC is less than twice that of the regular cycle interval. This is known as a *partial compensatory pause.* Since the PVC occurs between two consecutively conducted sinus beats, it is an *interpolated* PVC.

Premature Ventricular Contraction
No Pause

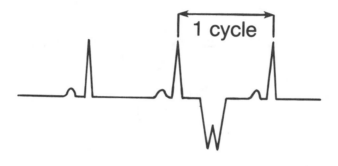

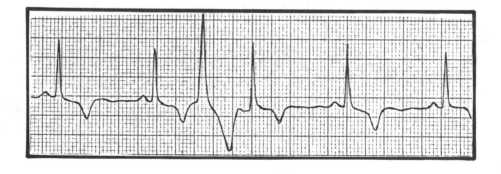

Less frequently, a PVC occurs without any pause. As illustrated above, the PVC does not interfere with the basic sinus rhythm. This PVC is also an interpolated PVC.

Premature Ventricular Contraction
Unifocal

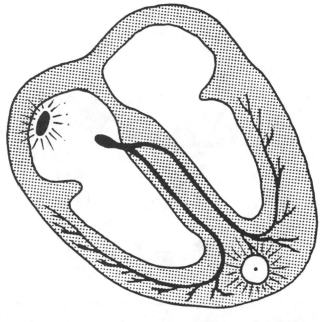

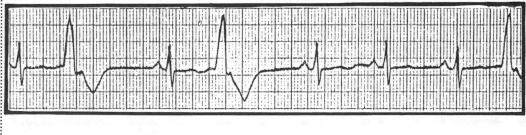

When all the PVCs originate in one focus, they are alike in configuration in any given lead. Note the relationship of each of the three PVCs to the preceding QRS complex. The distance between the preceding QRS complex and each PVC is identical. This is known as "fixed coupling" and is commonly seen.

Premature Ventricular Contractions
Multifocal

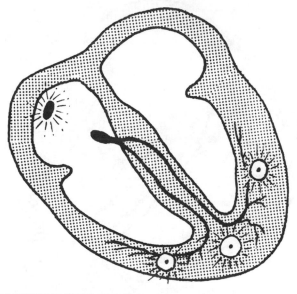

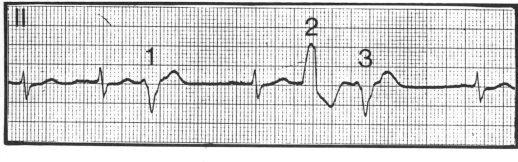

The three PVCs above originate in two foci. PVC 2 is different in configuration from PVCs 1 and 3. When PVCs originate in more than one focus, they are known as multifocal PVCs. The term "multiform" (or multiforme) has been recommended by some, since research has shown that PVCs of more than one configuration may originate in one focus.

Premature Ventricular Contractions

Couplets

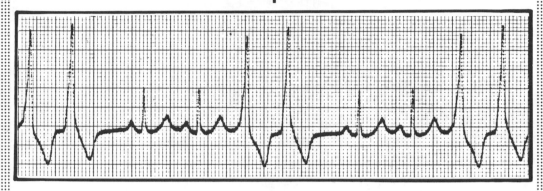

Salvo

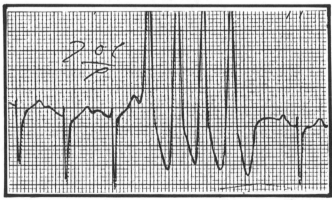

A *couplet* refers to two closely coupled PVCs in a row. A couplet should not be confused with the term coupling, which refers to the relationship of the PVC to the previous normal beat (see pp. 107 and 110).

A *salvo* is a run of three or more ventricular ectopic beats in a row. By definition, this is a burst of ventricular tachycardia.

Premature Ventricular Contractions
Bigeminy

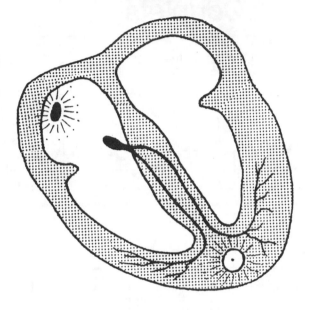

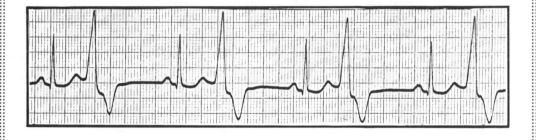

Bigeminy describes the heart beating in groups of two. In this patient, a normal beat is followed by a premature ventricular contraction and is separated from the next group by a pause. Trigeminy refers to heartbeats in groups of three. The words bigeminy and trigeminy do not reveal the components of the group; these must be described.

Premature Ventricular Contractions
"R-on-T" Phenomenon

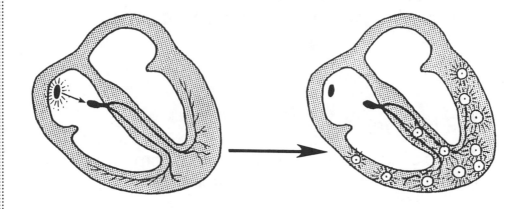

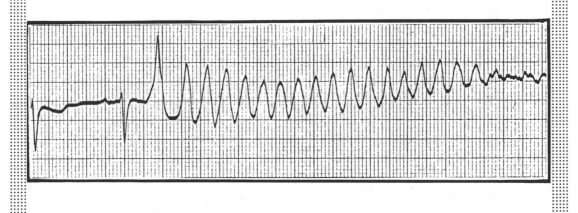

The *"R-on-T"* phenomenon refers to the close coupling of the premature beat with the preceding beat. Above we see the encroachment of the R wave of the PVC onto the T wave of the preceding beat. On p. 62 we differentiated between the absolute and relative refractory periods. The peak of the T wave is a vulnerable period, with the ability of a premature beat to initiate a dangerous arrhythmia. Here we see an "R-on-T" phenomenon setting off a catastrophic arrhythmia. The study of ventricular tachycardia, flutter and fibrillation is found on the next few pages.

Ventricular Tachycardia

1. P Wave:

P waves may not be distinguishable during ventricular tachycardia, although atrial activity, dissociated from ventricular activity, may not be affected.

2. PR Interval:

Since atrial activity is dissociated from ventricular activity, a PR interval is not measurable.

3. QRS Complex:

The QRS complex duration is greater than 0.12 sec., and bizarre in appearance. The T wave may not be separated from the QRS complex.

4. Rhythm:

The rhythm is regular or slightly irregular.

5. Rate:

The ventricular rate is 150 to 250 per minute. Atrial activity is often not determinable.

Ventricular Tachycardia
(Sustained)

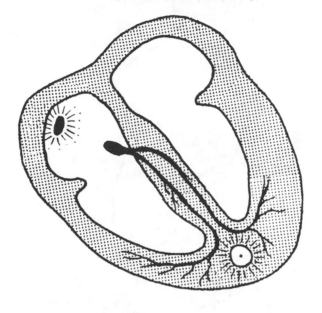

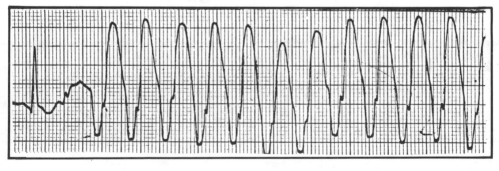

In *ventricular tachycardia* the ectopic pacemaker in the ventricle may produce "runs" of PVCs. Once started, ventricular tachycardia may be sustained until terminated spontaneously, by medication or by electrical cardioversion, or it may be intermittent. The QRS complexes are widened and bizarre, and the rate is usually from 150 to 250 beats per minute. The rhythm may be regular or slightly irregular. Atrial activity is usually not affected.

Ventricular Tachycardia
(Intermittent)

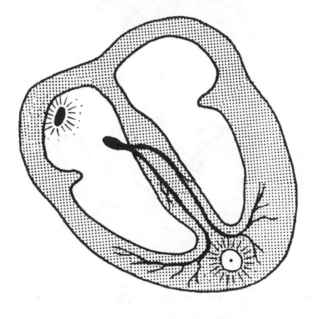

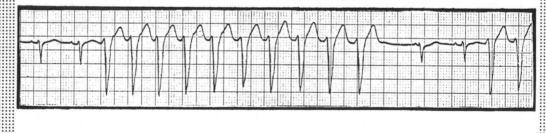

As noted on the previous page, ventricular tachycardia may be sustained or intermittent. Here, after two sinus beats, we see ten PVCs, a burst of ventricular tachycardia, then two more sinus beats followed by more PVCs.

Ventricular Tachycardia
(Torsade de Pointes)

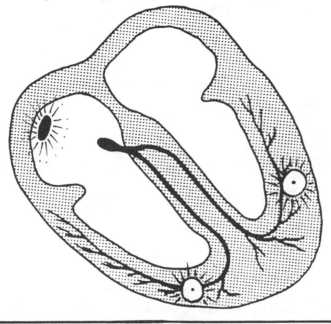

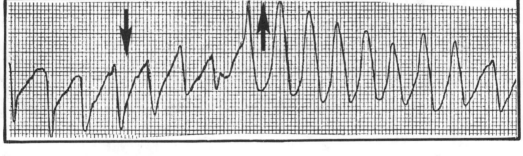

Ventricular tachycardia may be unifocal or multifocal. Periodically, in a given lead there are beats of one polarity followed by beats of the opposite polarity separated by beats of an intermediate form. This is known as torsade de pointes (turning of the points).

Accelerated Idioventricular Rhythm (AIVR)

1. P Wave:

P waves may not be distinguishable, as illustrated on p. 117.

2. PR Interval:

There is no measurable PR interval.

3. QRS Complex:

The QRS complex duration is usually 0.12 sec. or greater.

4. Rhythm:

The ventricular rhythm is regular or slightly irregular.

5. Rate:

The ventricular rate is 40 to 150 (usually 60-130) per minute and constant from beat to beat.

Accelerated Idioventricular Rhythm (AIVR)

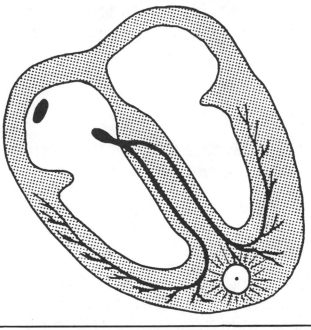

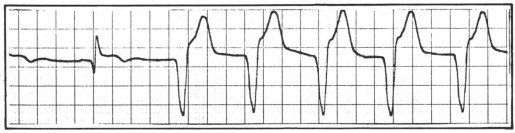

The accelerated idioventricular rhythm controls the heart at a rate from 40 to 150 (usually 60 to 130) beats per minute. This ectopic rhythm may be an "escape" or "safety" rhythm when the higher pacemakers begin to slow down or fail completely. It is commonly seen in patients with myocardial infarction. It very rarely progresses to a serious tachycardia and should not be suppressed.

Ventricular Flutter

1. P Wave:

P waves may not be distinguishable during ventricular flutter, although atrial activity, dissociated from ventricular activity, may not be affected.

2. PR Interval:

Since atrial activity is dissociated from ventricular activity, a PR interval is not measurable.

3. QRS Complex:

The QRS complex duration is greater than 0.12 sec., and bizarre in appearance. The T wave may not be separated from the QRS complex.

4. Rhythm:

The rhythm is regular or slightly irregular.

5. Rate:

The ventricular rate is 250 to 350 per minute. Atrial activity is often not determinable.

Ventricular Flutter

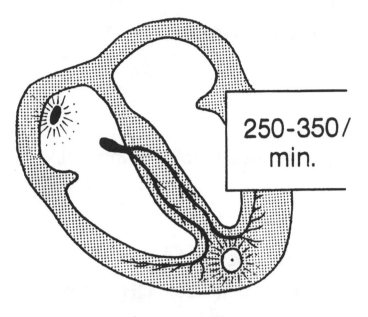

250-350/ min.

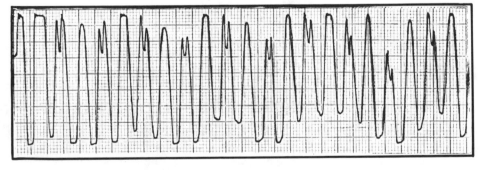

In *ventricular flutter*, undulating waves are seen rising and falling. This rhythm is often an intermediary stage between ventricular tachycardia and ventricular fibrillation. The rate is usually between 250 and 350 beats per minute. When the ventricular rate is at this level, the patient is acutely ill and the pulse may be imperceptible. The rate is too fast for ventricular tachycardia, which is usually about 160 beats per minute. The rhythm requires immediate interruption to sustain life. Atrial activity may be unaffected. The rhythm is usually short-lived, deteriorating into ventricular fibrillation within a very short time.

Ventricular Fibrillation

1. **P Wave:**

   P waves are not identifiable.

2. **PR Interval:**

   There is no measurable PR interval.

3. **QRS Complex:**

   There are no identifiable QRS complexes.

4. **Rhythm:**

   The rhythm is chaotic, with multiple, disorganized contractions of the ventricles.

5. **Rate:**

   The rate cannot be determined accurately.

Ventricular Fibrillation

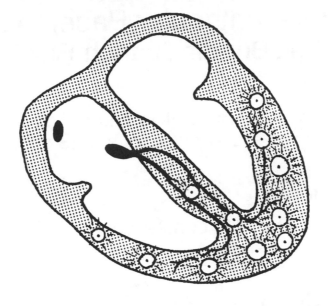

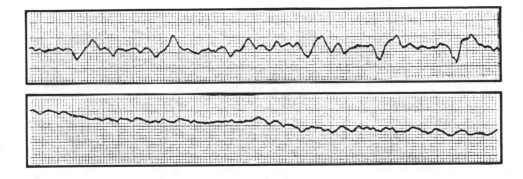

Multiple, disorganized contractions of the ventricles characterize *ventricular fibrillation* and represent *cardiac arrest*. It may be of sudden onset or may follow ventricular premature contractions, ventricular tachycardia and ventricular flutter. The immediate institution of cardiopulmonary resuscitation while waiting for electrical defibrillation may save the patient.

Wide QRS Complexes with Supraventricular Pacemaker
Left Bundle Branch Block

1. P Wave:

The P waves are positive and uniform in lead II. Every P wave is followed by a QRS complex.

2. PR Interval:

The PR interval is constant between 0.12 and 0.2 sec.

3. QRS Complex:

The QRS complex is abnormally wide, greater than 0.1 sec., and often greater than 0.12 sec. due to the intraventricular conduction disturbance (left bundle branch block, LBBB, p. 123). Every QRS complex is preceded by a P wave.

4. Rhythm:

The rhythm is regular.

5. Rate:

The rate, under the control of the SA node, is constant between 60 and 100 per minute.

Wide QRS Complexes With Supraventricular Pacemaker
Left Bundle Branch Block

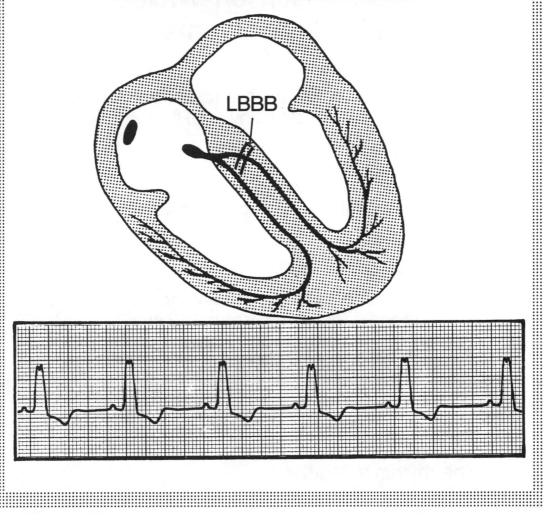

QRS Complex Width:

1. A normal narrow (up to 0.1 sec.) QRS complex indicates a supraventricular rhythm (sinus, atrial or junctional).

2. A ventricular rhythm has an abnormally wide QRS complex (usually wider than 0.12 sec.). See pp. 36, 98 and 99.

3. *An exception:* In the illustration above, we have all the requirements of normal sinus rhythm except that the QRS complex is wide (greater than 0.1 sec.). The rhythm is supraventricular, but since there is an *intraventricular conduction disturbance,* in this situation *left bundle branch block (LBBB)* with delayed ventricular depolarization, there is a wide QRS complex.

Wide QRS Complexes with Supraventricular Pacemaker Wolff-Parkinson-White (WPW) Syndrome

1. P Wave:

The P waves are positive and uniform in lead II. Every P wave is followed by a QRS complex.

2. PR Interval:

The PR interval is 0.12 sec. or less.

3. QRS Complex:

The QRS complex is abnormally wide, greater than 0.1 sec., and often greater than 0.12 sec. due to the slurred initial component known as the "delta" wave. Every QRS complex is preceded by a P wave.

4. Rhythm:

The rhythm is regular.

5. Rate:

The rate, under the control of the SA node, is constant between 60 and 100 per minute.

Wide QRS Complexes With Supraventricular Pacemaker Wolff-Parkinson-White (WPW)Syndrome

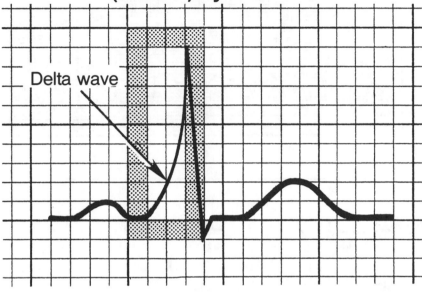

Delta wave

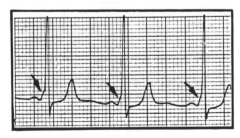

Another example of a wide QRS complex with a supraventricular pacemaker is the *Wolff-Parkinson-White (WPW) syndrome.* The WPW syndrome represents an anomalous pathway or bypass from the atria to the ventricles. Because patients with the syndrome may be subject to attacks of paroxysmal tachycardia, it is included in the study of arrhythmias. The electrocardiographic characteristics include:

1. Short PR interval (0.12 sec. or less).
2. Prolonged QRS interval (greater than 0.1 sec.).
3. Slurring of the upstroke by a *delta* wave.

Practice
Rhythm Analysis

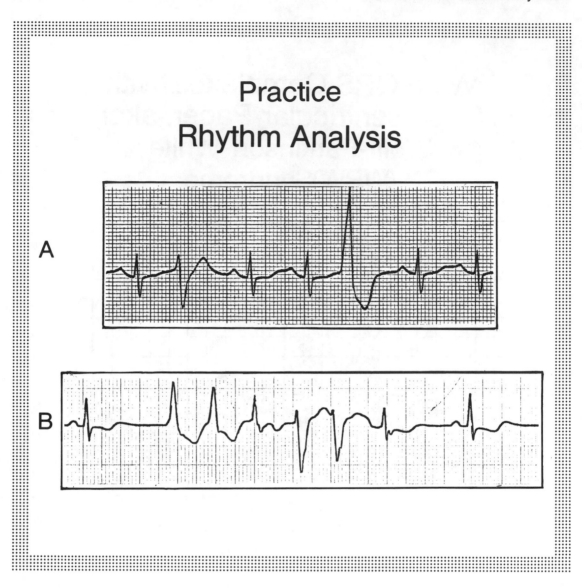

Analysis A: **Analysis B:**

RHYTHM ANALYSIS

A. 1. P Wave:
   The P waves of the underlying basic rhythm are positive. The two ectopic beats are not preceded by P waves.

2. PR Interval:
   The PR interval of the basic rhythm is 0.2 sec.

3. QRS Complex:
   The QRS complex duration in the basic rhythm is 0.08 sec. Whereas in the ectopic beats the QRS complexes are 0.16 sec. and 0.12 sec., respectively.

4. Rhythm:
   The rhythm is irregular. The regularity of the basic rhythm is disturbed by the ectopic beats.

5. Rate:
   The basic rate is 103 beats per minute.

Impression and Comment:

Sinus tachycardia with multifocal PVCs. The term "multiform" instead of "multifocal" has been recommended by some because research has shown that PVCs of more than one configuration may originate in one focus.

B. 1. P Wave:
   The P waves of the underlying basic rhythm are positive and uniform. The ectopic beats are not preceded by P waves.

2. PR Interval:
   The PR interval of the basic rhythm is 0.18 sec. Since there are no P waves associated with the wide QRS complexes, there are no measurable PR intervals.

3. QRS Complex:
   The QRS complex duration of the basic rhythm is 0.08 sec. The QRS complex duration of the ectopic beats is 0.14 sec. These QRS complexes consist of complexes of opposite polarity. The first two complexes are positive, followed by an intermediate form and then by negative complexes.

4. Rhythm:
   The regularity of the basic rhythm is disturbed by a group of ectopic beats.

5. Rate:
   The rate of the ectopic rhythm is 150 beats per minute. The rate of the basic rhythm cannot be determined because we do not have two consecutive normal beats.

Impression and Comment:

Sinus rhythm with a run of Ventricular Tachycardia, multifocal. The two groups of ectopic QRS complexes of opposite polarity are separated by an intermediate form. This is known as torsade de pointes.

Chapter 7

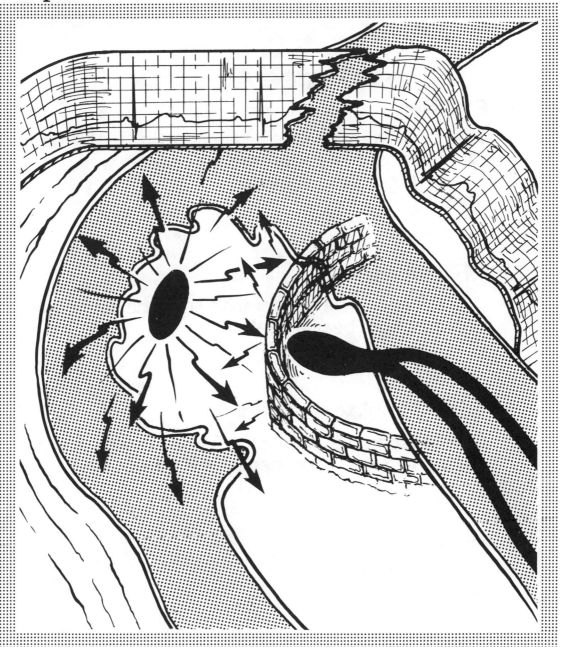

Atrioventricular (AV) Conduction Disturbances

First Degree AV Block
Second Degree AV Block
Wenckebach Block
(Mobitz I Block)

Mobitz II Block
Third Degree (Complete)
AV Block
Pacemaker Therapy

First Degree AV Block

1. P Wave:

The P waves are positive and uniform in lead II if the SA node is the pacemaker. Every P wave is followed by a QRS complex.

2. PR Interval:

The PR interval is greater than 0.12 sec. and constant from beat to beat.

3. QRS Complex:

The QRS complex duration is 0.1 sec. or less. Every QRS complex is preceded by a P wave.

4. Rhythm:

The rhythm is regular.

5. Rate:

The rate is dependent on the basic rhythm. If the basic rhythm is sinus, the rate is constant between 60 and 100 per minute.

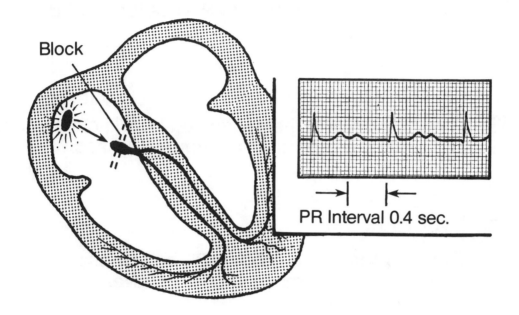

First Degree AV Block

Block

PR Interval 0.4 sec.

Prolongation of PR Interval
>0.2 sec.

First degree atrioventricular (AV) block represents a delay in the transmission of impulses from the atria to the ventricles. The delay commonly occurs in the AV node but may occur below it. *A prolonged PR interval (greater than 0.2 sec.)* is seen on this electrocardiogram.

Second Degree AV Block

1. P Wave:

    The P waves are positive and uniform in con-figuration in lead II. Not every P wave is followed by a QRS complex.

2. PR Interval:

    The PR interval of the conducted beat is constant and may be greater than the normal 0.2 sec.

3. QRS Complex:

    The QRS complex duration is 0.1 sec. or less. Every QRS complex is preceded by a P wave.

4. Rhythm:

    The rhythm is regular when there is a stable atrial to ventricular relationship, e.g., 2:1, 3:1. If this relation-ship varies, the rhythm is irregular.

5. Rate:

    Because of the AV block, the atrial rate is often two, three or four times that of the ventricular rate.

Second Degree AV Block

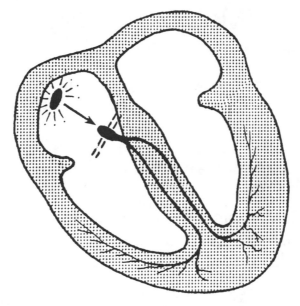

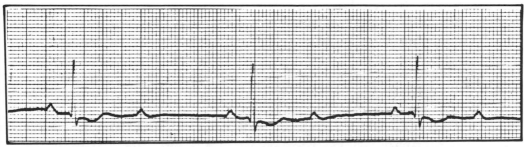

2:1 AV Block

When the ventricles do not respond to atrial stimuli, the P wave is not followed by a QRS complex. The various grades of *second degree AV block* are recognized by the frequency and characteristics of blocked atrial conduction. Seen above are two atrial deflections for every ventricular deflection, or 2:1 AV block. The atrial rate is 62 and the ventricular rate is 31 beats per minute. Three and four P waves for every QRS complex would be known as 3:1 and 4:1 AV block, respectively.

Second Degree AV Block
(Wenckebach Block)
(Mobitz I Block)

1. P Wave:

   The P waves are positive and uniform in lead II. Not every P wave is followed by a QRS complex.

2. PR Interval:

   The PR intervals become progressively longer until an atrial depolarization no longer initiates a ventricular response. The cycle is then resumed.

3. QRS Complex:

   The QRS complex duration is 0.1 sec. or less.

4. Rhythm:

   The rhythm is irregular with "grouped beating." As illustrated on p. 135, there is a pause after each group of three ventricular beats.

5. Rate:

   The atrial rate is constant between 60 and 100 per minute. The ventricular rate is slower due to the nonconducted beats.

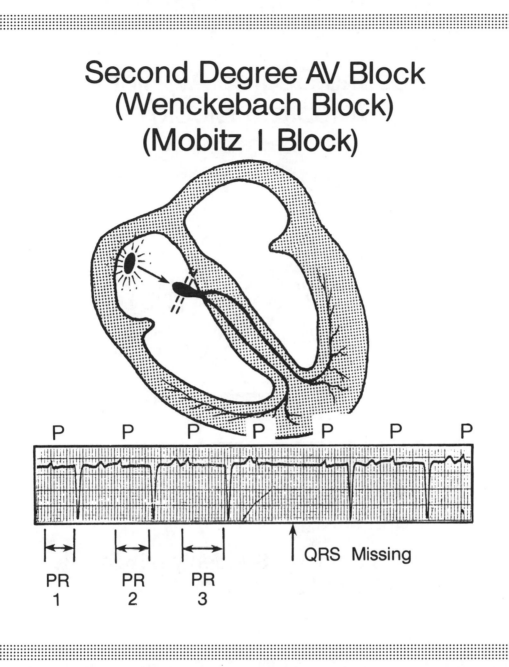

Second Degree AV Block
(Wenckebach Block)
(Mobitz I Block)

P P P P P P P

PR 1   PR 2   PR 3   ↑ QRS Missing

In Mobitz I block ventricular beats are "dropped" in a cyclic manner. The PR interval is less prolonged at first but becomes progressively longer, until an atrial contraction no longer initiates a ventricular response. The cycle is then resumed. In the above electrocardiogram, the first PR interval is shorter than the second, which is shorter than the third. The fourth P wave does not conduct and is therefore not followed by a QRS complex. The fifth P wave starts the cycle again.

Second Degree AV Block
(Mobitz II Block)

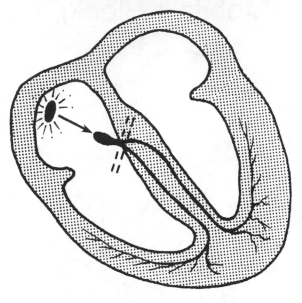

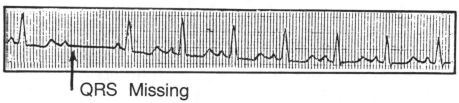

↑ QRS Missing

1. QRS Complex Suddenly Missing
2. PR Intervals Unchanged

Mobitz II block is classified under second AV block, since P waves are periodically not followed by QRS complexes (arrow). Electrophysiologic studies have shown that the site of block is usually below the AV node and may be a warning of future complete AV block.

Second Degree AV Block

A
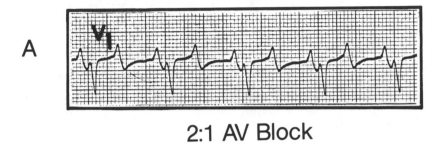

2:1 AV Block

B
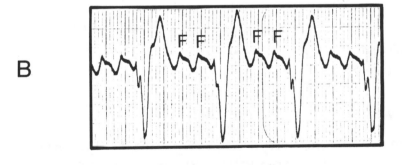

4:1 AV Block

Above are two and four atrial deflections (P waves or flutter waves) for every ventricular deflection (QRS complex), respectively. Conduction ratios, e.g., 2:1 and 4:1, should not be emphasized at the expense of rate. A conduction ratio of 2:1, as in the example on p. 133, with an atrial rate of 62 and a dangerously low ventricular rate of 31, is in sharp contrast with (A) and (B) above. Here atrial rates of 150 and 300 result in ventricular rates of 75 with conduction ratios of 2:1 and 4:1. In these two cases, the AV node is actually protecting the heart by not allowing every impulse to be transmitted to the ventricles.

Third Degree (Complete) AV Block

1. P Wave:

The P waves are positive and uniform in lead II and are not associated with the QRS complexes.

2. PR Interval:

Since there is no relationship between the P waves and the QRS complexes, there is no measurable PR interval.

3. QRS Complex:

The QRS complex duration, depending on the site of impulse formation, may be normal, as on p. 139, with the pacemaker in the AV junction, or quite wide and bizarre, with the pacemaker low in the ventricles.

4. Rhythm:

The ventricular rhythm is regular. The atrial rhythm will depend on the intrinsic atrial pacemaker.

5. Rate:

The atria are often controlled by the SA node while the venticles are controlled by either a junctional pacemaker with a normally narrow QRS complex or a ventricular pacemaker with a wide, bizarre QRS complex.

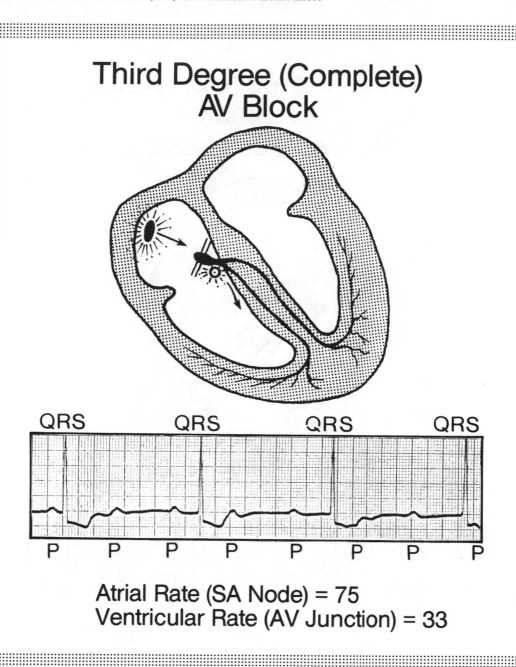

Third Degree (Complete) AV Block

QRS   QRS   QRS   QRS

P   P   P   P   P   P   P   P

Atrial Rate (SA Node) = 75
Ventricular Rate (AV Junction) = 33

In *third degree,* or *complete AV block,* there is no relationship between the atria and the ventricles. The atria, remaining under the control of the SA node, are beating at 75 per minute and are completely dissociated from the ventricles. Depending on the site of impulse formation, the QRS complexes may be of normal duration, as above, with the pacemaker in the AV junction, or quite wide and bizarre, with the pacemaker low in the ventricles. The ventricular rate is 33 beats per minute.

Third Degree (Complete) AV Block Pacemaker Therapy

Pacemaker

Pacemaker Impulses

I   II   III

A patient with complete AV block, as seen here, may present with symptoms of cerebral insufficiency, such as dizziness or clouded mentation, or may actually have lost consciousness (Adams-Stokes syndrome) as a result of the low heart rate and poor cardiac output or of transient ventricular standstill or fibrillation. The present-day treatment is electrical pacing to maintain a proper rate and good cardiac output. The arrows point to pacemaker impulses.

Practice
Rhythm Analysis

Practice
Rhythm Analysis

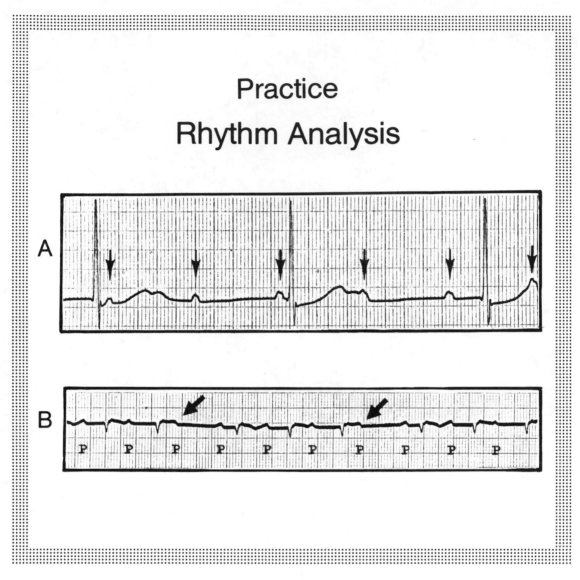

Analysis A:

Analysis B:

RHYTHM ANALYSIS

A. 1. P Wave:
    The P waves (arrows) are positive and uniform and are not associated with the QRS complexes.
  2. PR Interval:
    Since there is no relationship between the P waves and the QRS complexes, there is no measurable PR interval.
  3. QRS Complex:
    The QRS complex duration is 0.08 sec.
  4. Rhythm:
    The rhythm is regular (both atrial and ventricular), since both the atria and ventricles are responding to their own separate pacemakers.
  5. Rate:
    The atrial rate is 68 beats per minute and the ventricular rate is 29 beats per minute.

Impression and Comment:

Third Degree (Complete) AV Block. The atria are under the control of the SA node, whereas the ventricles are under the control of the AV junction.

B. 1. P Wave:
    The P waves are positive and uniform. Not every P wave is followed by a QRS complex. The arrows point to the P waves not followed by QRS complexes.
  2. PR Interval:
    The PR intervals become progressively longer until an atrial depolarization no longer initiates a ventricular response. The cycle is then resumed.
  3. QRS Complex:
    The QRS complex duration is 0.06 sec.
  4. Rhythm:
    The rhythm is irregular with "grouped beating." There is a pause after each group of three ventricular beats.
  5. Rate:
    The atrial rate is 100 beats per minute, and the average ventricular rate is 80 beats per minute.

Impression and Comment:

Second Degree AV Block (Wenckebach or Mobitz I Block). The ventricular rate is slower due to the nonconducted beats. The AV conduction ratio is 4:3, four atrial beats for every three ventricular beats.

Additional Rhythm Analyses
for
Practice and Review

Practice
Rhythm Analysis

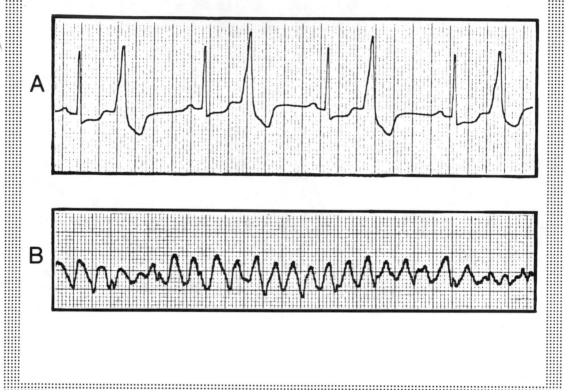

Analysis A: **Analysis B:**

RHYTHM ANALYSIS

A. 1. P Wave:
   The P waves preceding the QRS complexes of the underlying basic rhythm are positive and uniform. There are no P waves associated with the wide ectopic QRS complexes.
   2. PR Interval:
   The PR interval of the basic rhythm is 0.2 sec.
   3. QRS Complex:
   The QRS complex duration of the basic rhythm is 0.08 sec. The ectopic QRS complex duration is 0.16 sec.
   4. Rhythm:
   The rhythm is irregular, with beats in groups of two forming a bigeminal rhythm. Each ectopic beat is coupled with a normal beat.
   5. Rate:
   The rate of the basic rhythm measures 44 beats per minute. Most likely, there is a P wave hidden within the ectopic QRS complex, not seen on the electrocardiogram, resulting in a basic rate of 88 beats per minute.

Impression and Comment:

Sinus Rhythm with unifocal fixed coupled PVCs in bigeminy. The term bigeminy does not reveal the components of each group of two. It only refers to the heart beating in groups of two; these must be described. In this particular case, the true sinus rate is not known. The rate could be 44 or 88 beats per minute. If the latter is the situation, the nonconducted P waves are completely hidden within the ectopic complex. (See pages 107 and 110.)

B. 1. P Wave:
   No P waves are identifiable.
   2. PR Interval:
   There is no measurable PR interval.
   3. QRS Complex:
   There are no identifiable QRS complexes.
   4. Rhythm:
   The rhythm is chaotic with multiple disorganized contractions of the ventricles.
   5. Rate:
   The rate cannot be accurately determined.

Impression and Comment:

Ventricular Fibrillation. This arrhythmia represents cardiac arrest. (See pages 120 and 121.)

Practice
Rhythm Analysis

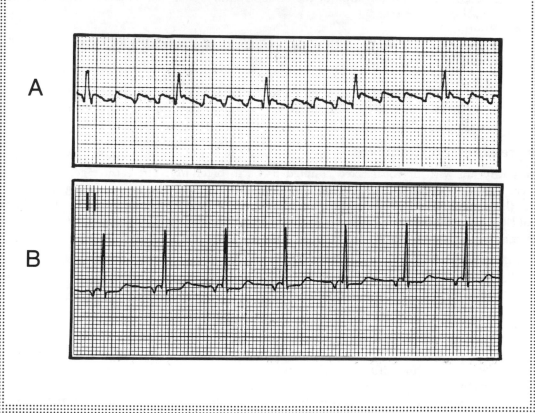

Analysis A: **Analysis B:**

RHYTHM ANALYSIS

A. 1. P Wave:
The atrial deflections, with a saw-tooth appearance, are known as flutter waves.
2. PR Interval:
Because of the characteristic appearance of the flutter waves, it is often difficult to determine the PR interval. It is, therefore, not measured.
3. QRS Complex:
The QRS complex duration is 0.08 sec.
4. Rhythm:
The rhythm is regular, with a 4:1 conduction ratio (four atrial beats for every ventricular beat).
5. Rate:
The atrial rate is 260 and the ventricular rate is 65 beats per minute.

Impression and Comment:

Atrial Flutter with a 4:1 conduction ratio. (See pages 66, 67, and 137.) The AV node is protecting the heart by permitting only one of four atrial impulses to be transmitted to the ventricles.

B. 1. P Wave:
An inverted P wave precedes each QRS complex in lead II.
2. PR Interval:
The PR interval is 0.12 sec.
3. QRS Complex:
The QRS complex duration is 0.07 sec.
4. Rhythm:
The rhythm is regular.
5. Rate:
The rate is constant at 94 beats per minute.

Impression and Comment:

Accelerated Junctional Rhythm. All the characteristics of junctional rhythm are met except rate. (See pages 88 and 89.)

Practice
Rhythm Analysis

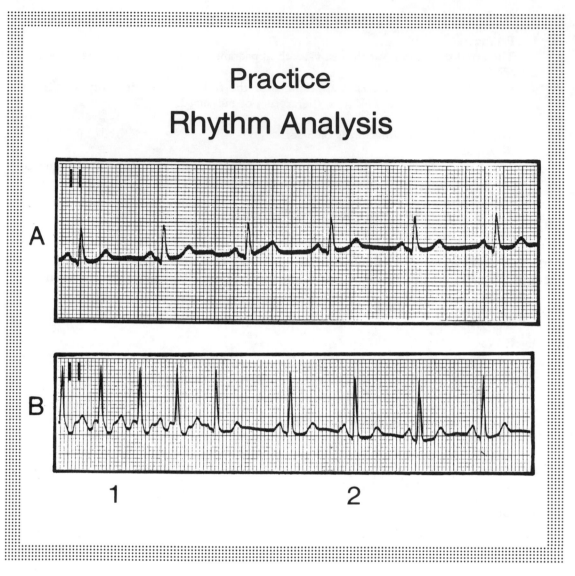

Analysis A: **Analysis B:**

RHYTHM ANALYSIS

A. 1. P Wave:
   The P waves are positive and uniform in lead II. Every P wave is followed by a QRS complex.
   2. PR Interval:
   The PR interval is 0.16 sec.
   3. QRS Complex:
   The QRS complex duration is 0.08 sec. Every QRS complex is preceded by a P wave.
   4. Rhythm:
   The rhythm is regular.
   5. Rate:
   The rate is 70 beats per minute.

Impression and Comment:

Normal Sinus Rhythm. (See pages 42 and 43.)

B. 1. P Wave:
   The atrial deflections in rhythm 1, with a saw-tooth appearance, are known as flutter waves. The P waves in rhythm 2 are positive and uniform in lead II, and every P wave is followed by a QRS complex.
   2. PR Interval:
   In rhythm 1, because the characteristic appearance of the flutter waves, it is often difficult to determine the PR interval. It is therefore, not measured. In rhythm 2 the PR interval is 0.16 sec.
   3. QRS Complex:
   The QRS complex duration is 0.06 sec. In rhythm 2 every QRS complex is preceded by a P wave.
   4. Rhythm:
   Rhythm 1 is regular, with a 2:1 conduction ratio (two atrial beats for every ventricular beat). Rhythm 2 is regular.
   5. Rate:
   In rhythm 1, the atrial rate is 300 and the ventricular rate is 150 beats per minute. In rhythm 2 the rate is 88 beats per minute.

Impression and Comment:

Atrial Flutter (rhythm 1) converting spontaneously to Normal Sinus Rhythm (rhythm 2). Note the slight pause between the two rhythms. (See pages 66 and 67.)

Practice
Rhythm Analysis

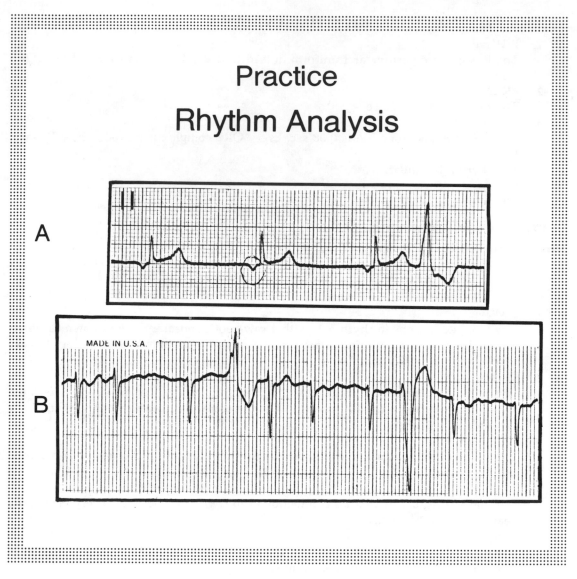

Analysis A:

Analysis B:

RHYTHM ANALYSIS

A. 1. P Wave:
The P waves preceding the QRS complexes in the basic rhythm are inverted in lead II. There is no P wave associated with the ectopic QRS complex.

2. PR Interval:
The PR interval of the basic rhythm is 0.12 sec.

3. QRS Complex:
The QRS complex duration of the basic rhythm is 0.06 sec. and that of the ectopic beat is 0.14 sec.

4. Rhythm:
The very slight irregularity of the basic rhythm is disturbed by an ectopic beat.

5. Rate:
The rate of the basic rhythm is 52 beats per minute.

Impression and Comment:

Junctional Rhythm with a PVC. The intrinsic rate of the junctional pacemaker is 40 to 60 beats per minute. (See pages 80 and 81, 102 and 103.)

B. 1. P Wave:
There are no identifiable P waves, only fibrillatory waves, irregular movements of the baseline.

2. PR Interval:
Since there are no identifiable P waves, there is no measurable PR interval.

3. QRS Complex:
The QRS complex duration in the basic rhythm is 0.08 sec. Those of the ectopic beats are 0.12 sec. and 0.16 sec., respectively. The two ectopic beats are of different configurations.

4. Rhythm:
The rhythm is irregularly irregular and is further disturbed by ectopic beats.

5. Rate:
The atrial rate is above 300 with a chaotic rhythm. The ventricular rate is 100 beats per minute (average).

Impression and Comment:

Atrial Fibrillation with multifocal PVCs and a ventricular response of 100 beats per minute. There is no stable relationship between the fibrillatory atrial waves and the QRS complexes. Most of the atrial impulses are blocked in the AV node. (See pages 68 and 69, 102 and 103, and 108.)

Practice
Rhythm Analysis

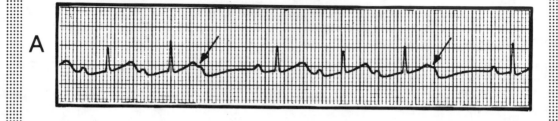

A

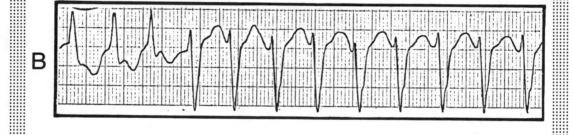

B

Analysis A: **Analysis B:**

RHYTHM ANALYSIS

A. 1. P Wave:

The P waves are positive. Not every P wave is followed by a QRS complex. The arrows point to the P waves, which are not followed by QRS complexes.

2. PR Interval:

The PR intervals become progressively longer until an atrial depolarization no longer initiates a ventricular response. The cycle is then resumed.

3. QRS Complex:

The QRS complex duration is 0.06 sec.

4. Rhythm:

The rhythm is irregular, with "grouped beating." There is a pause after each group of three ventricular beats.

5. Rate:

The atrial rate is 95 beats per minute, and the average ventricular rate is 73 beats per minute.

Impression and Comment:

Second Degree AV Block (Wenckebach or Mobitz I Block). (See pages 134 and 135.) The ventricular rate is lower than the atrial rate due to the nonconducted beats. The AV conduction ratio is 4:3, four atrial beats for every three ventricular beats.

B. 1. P Wave:

P waves are not clearly identifiable.

2. PR Interval:

Since P waves are not identifiable, there is no measurable PR interval.

3. QRS Complex:

The QRS complex duration is 0.14 sec. The QRS complexes consist of beats of opposite polarity. The first two complexes are positive, followed by an intermediate form and then negative complexes.

4. Rhythm:

The rhythm is slightly irregular.

5. Rate:

The rate is 140 beats per minute.

Impression and Comment:

Ventricular Tachycardia, multifocal. The groups of QRS complexes of opposite polarity (separated by an intermediate form) are known as torsade de pointes. P waves may not be distinguishable during ventricular tachycardia, although atrial activity, dissociated from ventricular activity, may not be affected. (See pages 112, 113, and 115.)

Practice
Rhythm Analysis

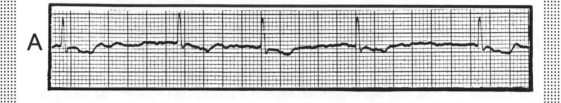

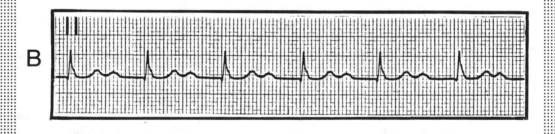

Analysis A: **Analysis B:**

RHYTHM ANALYSIS

A. 1. P Wave:

   There are no identifiable P waves, only fibrillatory waves, irregular movements of the baseline.

   2. PR Interval:

   Since there are no identifiable P waves, there is no measurable PR interval.

   3. QRS Complex:

   The QRS complex duration is 0.08 sec.

   4. Rhythm:

   The rhythm is irregular.

   5. Rate:

   The atrial rate is above 350 beats per minute with a chaotic rhythm. The ventricular response is irregular with an average rate of 55 beats per minute.

Impression and Comment:

Atrial Fibrillation with a slow ventricular response of 55 beats per minute. There is no stable relationship between the fibrillatory atrial waves and the QRS complexes. Most of the atrial impulses are blocked at the AV node. (See pages 68 and 69.)

B. 1. P Wave:

   The P waves are positive and uniform in lead II. Every P wave is followed by a QRS complex.

   2. PR Interval:

   The PR interval is 0.4 sec.

   3. QRS Complex:

   The QRS complex duration is 0.1 sec. Every QRS complex is preceded by a P wave.

   4. Rhythm:

   The rhythm is regular.

   5. Rate:

   The rate is 75 beats per minute.

Impression and Comment:

Sinus Rhythm with First Degree AV Block. First degree AV block represents a delay in the transmission of impulses from the atria to ventricles. The delay commonly occurs in the AV node but may occur below it. (See pages 130 and 131.)

INDEX